UNL[OCK]
YOUR [MIND]
AND BE
FREE!

A Practical Approach to Hypnotherapy

Edgar A. Barnett M.D.

Published by WESTWOOD PUBLISHING COMPANY
700 S. CENTRAL AVENUE, GLENDALE, CA 91204
(818)242-1159

For catalog of HYPNOTISM and MIND
POWER Books, Cassettes and
Videocassettes write to:

WESTWOOD PUBLISHING CO.
700 S. CENTRAL AVENUE
GLENDALE, CA 91024
(818)242-1159

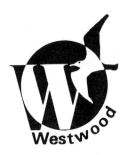

ISBN 0-930298-49-7
Library of Congress Catalog Card Number 79-87715

PREFACE

Twenty years ago, Dr. Edgar Barnett was a traditional general practitioner who found the illnesses of some of his patients couldn't be helped by traditional medicines and therapies because many had a deeply hidden emotional basis. He began using hypnosis and found it so successful that he now practices exclusively as a hypnotherapist in Kingston, Ont. His book on hypnoanalysis is far more thought-provoking than the title suggests; in all Barnett likens the troubled person to a prisoner locked in the cell of his or her own mind. Hypnosis can be the key to unlocking it as patients enter their subconscious and with skillful guidance recognize, accept and attempt to solve emotional difficulties. Barnett's case studies are fascinating, his ideas surprisingly uplifting; there's also a section on self-hypnosis and self-analysis.

In his exciting new book, Dr. Barnett discusses the use of hypnotic regression which allows his patient's subconscious to seek out the traumatic emotional experiences which are directly responsible for their present difficulties. He verifies that even at the moment of birth a newborn can hear and emotionally respond to such statements as, "I never wanted this baby!" or "But I wanted a boy!"

Your medical and scientific library will be enhanced by Dr. Barnett's book.

An extraordinary conceptualization of a system of hypnotherapy that is not only unique but amazingly effective. I give this book a 5-star rating. A must for the serious-minded hypnotherapist.

Gil Boyne, certified Hypnotherapist
Exec. Dir. **American Council of Hypnotist Examiners**
Pres. **Hypnotist Examining Council of California**

DEDICATION

To Margaret
Carolyn, Nigel and Judith

CONTENTS

ACKNOWLEDGMENTS

The encouragement to write this book came from fellow hypnotherapists and friends whose faith in my ability to accomplish this task was matched by their belief that it would meet a popular need to understand the principles and aims of hypnoanalysis.

Fellow Canadian hypnoanalysts, Dr. David Craig and Dr. Daniel Stewart provided constant support and advice throughout this venture and my dear friend Dr. Edith Fiore, gave freely of her valuable experience and wisdom during the early stages of the preparation of the manuscript.

It is to Dr. David Cheek of San Francisco that I owe my commitment to hypnoanalysis as a valid approach to therapy for it is from his workshops, seminars and writings that I have been able to fashion the tools to discover the material within this book.

My thanks go also to Mr. John Cruickshanks and Mrs. Bonnie Kellar for their invaluable help in the editing and preparation of the original manuscript.

For each of the three patients whose experience of hypnoanalysis has been recorded in detail I have a special feeling of gratitude since they, as with the many patients whose stories I have used in an unrecognizable way, have made a valuable contribution to an understanding of this therapy.

INTRODUCTION

When I took up the general practice of medicine thirty years ago, it was widely believed that the profession was making great strides towards subduing many of mankind's most frightening illnesses. Penicillin and related antibiotics were revolutionizing the treatment of diseases. Pneumonia, once a menacing killer, was now under control. Polio would soon be vanquished by vaccine.

But after several years of working in a full and varied practice, I became aware that many of our hopes were ill-founded. The wonder drugs remained powerless against a large proportion of the illnesses a family practitioner faced. I soon realized that I had a poor understanding of the causes which underlay numerous maladies afflicting my patients, and none of my medical books carried any effective remedies.

During any one morning I treated patients with recurring headaches, muscle pains and vague feelings of discomfort. In time I learned that the presence of these symptoms did not necessarily indicate any discoverable disease of the kind that I had been trained to detect. Medicine geared to deal exclusively with physical complaints was failing these sufferers.

In my early years I became familiar with another variety of disorders which were periodic in nature, primarily occurring when patients experienced abnormal tensions in their lives. But it was always difficult to discover why these patients who were suffering from such poorly understood disorders as ulcers, high blood pressure, migraine and asthma would recover quickly on some occasions and respond slowly to treatment on others.

Then there were the frankly psychiatric problems for which the term "nervous breakdown" was, and still is, frequently used. These people were extremely tense or depressed, often erratic and unpredictable in their behavior.

Lacking the time in a busy general practice to provide adequate attention to patients with psychiatric problems, I referred them to psychiatrists in the belief that with a specialist they would receive the assistance necessary for recovery. To my dismay, it soon became clear that the psychiatrists made real and permanent progress with few of these patients, their greatest successes arising among those who were receptive to the kind and close attention which, but for the want of time, I would have been able to administer myself.

During this period psychotropic drugs became widely available and promised to revolutionize the treatment of emotional disorders in the way that antibiotics had transformed organic medicine. Valium, librium and other tranquilizers in varying strengths were useful in sedating patients, making them more manageable and receptive to treatment. But the psychotropics failed to live up to their early promise. They alleviated the symptoms of emotional distress without addressing the causes. The real problem of developing a cure for emotional illness remained.

Frustrated by the failure of psychotropics and conventional medical practices, I became convinced that a more personalized therapy which allowed the sufferer to deal constructively with his own problems must be found. In search of a form of therapy which could provide individual answers to individual problems, some twenty years ago I began to use hypnosis in my practice.

I first became interested in hypnosis as a young boy and from that time onward read every treatise I could obtain on the subject. I learned that mere suggestion in hypnosis could make the paralyzed walk and cure the asthmatic's wheeze. I read that mothers could deliver babies painlessly without anesthesia and that a wide variety of ills which apparently stemmed from organic causes could be defeated through the power of hypnosis. But my colleagues scoffed at these notions, and I remained uncertain as to the true value of such a therapy.

My interest in the power of suggestion continued unabated, and when I discovered that anyone could become proficient in the practice of hypnosis, I began to wonder whether it might provide fresh answers to the old problems I faced in my practice. It was not, however, until a patient suffering from a recurring migraine asked me if there was nothing else I could do for her that I suggested hypnosis.

My patient, naturally, was surprised by the suggestion that hypnosis might provide the key for her cure and was even more astounded to learn that I proposed to administer treatment myself. But she assented to the experiment, little knowing that I was a novice. I determined to conceal the fact until we could assess the results of the treatment, certain that success would be more likely if her confidence in me were maintained.

My first experience with hypnosis proved to be an unqualified success, for my patient made significant improvement. Her migraines, which had responded only temporarily to drug therapy, diminished in frequency and severity. She began to sleep more easily, and her emotional symptoms of depression and anxiety became much less pronounced. To conclude the treatment, I taught her how to induce self-hypnosis, and she was eventually able to discontinue the use of all the medications upon which she relied.

Naturally, I was highly impressed by this initial victory, and over the years I gradually increased my use of hypnosis. Simply by learning a process to aid relaxation, many of my patients were saved years of misery from tension induced complaints. But some of my patients had much more serious and complex problems.

Increased experience with hypnosis brought me greater insight into the underlying causes of deep-seated emotional distress. Patients whose complaints were obviously serious revealed to me a chilling degree of self-hatred. They craved relief but were unable to escape self-destructive patterns of behavior. Their physical symptoms were not the result of any organic disease but of emotional problems to which they were indissolubly tied. They had lost their freedom and their hope because they hadn't even realized they were imprisoned.

After almost three decades in hospital and family practice, I resolved to devote the remainder of my medical life solely to the practice of therapy through hypnosis. I had explored and appreciated the value of direct suggestion in hypnosis, but I have come to realize that its analytical powers give far superior results. In my experience hypnoanalysis has provided the most dependable key for unlocking the spirits and bodies of those who are shackled in the prisons of the mind.

Through the use of hypnoanalytic techniques I have had considerable success in helping patients discover the critical experiences in their backgrounds which have been responsible for their distress. The procedures I have developed, allowing patients to understand the importance of these critical experiences, have led to cures which would have been impossible with the use of hypnotic suggestion alone.

I have written this book in order to present my understanding of the conflicts which imprison us and of the means by which hypnoanalytic techniques can be used to find freedom.

I present these ideas so that you too can unlock your mind and be free.

Chapter One

Prisons Of The Mind

1. The Prison of Fear
Phobias

In the early years of my hypnotherapy practice, a young man came to me with a problem that was rapidly destroying his career. He had heard of my success with hypnosis and requested a consultation since all other measures to find a cure had failed.

"I'm a salesman, doctor, so I'm on the road a good deal. I like the work, and it's been going very well until recently. I've just started bringing in bonus money, but now . . . now my nerve seems to be failing," he said with a weak attempt at a grin.

George was a rugged, good-looking fellow of about thirty. He had worked as a laborer for several years, traveling whenever the spirit moved him. He had then married and settled down to a career in sales. A strong, independent individual, he could hardly admit to himself that he harbored a serious problem.

"I don't know where to start. It sounds so stupid. I just can't understand why this is happening to me. When I'm driving, I get a panicky feeling. I feel as if I'm going to swerve into the oncoming traffic. When this sensation comes over me, I start to shake. It gets so bad now that I have to pull off the road and calm down. I can't drive any faster than forty miles an hour on the highways anymore. I'm terrified. Because I keep having to stop, I'm late for every appointment I make, and my customers are beginning to think I'm unreliable. My boss is upset. Even my wife is wondering about me. I can't possibly go on like this."

It cost George considerable effort to tell his story. By the end he was sweating heavily and grimacing in emotional distress. I encouraged him to relax, assured him that my practice had made me familiar with problems of this kind, and began to question him about his terrifying experiences.

"How long have you been having these attacks George?" I asked.

"They began about three years ago. I didn't tell anybody. I didn't want anybody to know. They weren't as bad then, and they only happened once in a while. Now they occur almost any time I'm in the car."

"Do you ever get these attacks at other times when you're not driving?" I queried.

"No . . . ah, yes, but just once, a couple of weeks ago. I was up on the roof of the house trying to fix the TV antenna—just about 10 feet off the ground. I've never been afraid of heights, but up there I got the terrible feeling that I was going to leap off and smash myself on the ground. I took a few deep breaths and came down slowly, but the experience shook me up. It was so dumb but so frightening."

When George finished outlining his symptoms, I explained to him that he had developed a phobia.

"George, you must first understand that there's nothing stupid or dumb about what you're going through. This fear is very real for you. In fact, fear is like a prison. If you don't try to break out when it has locked you in, you'll never be a free man again—free to live your life the way you want to.

"Phobias are not really uncommon; many people suffer from them. You probably know somebody with an unnatural fear of snakes or heights or elevators . . . something like that. It seems silly on the outside, but those people feel the same kind of terror that you do about driving. Now this may be a little difficult to understand, but I don't think you're really afraid of driving, George."

"But doctor, it's so real."

"I don't doubt that, but were you ever afraid of driving three years ago?" I asked.

"No, never," he assured me.

"What's happened, George, is that you've developed a deeper fear within. Driving the car is just the trigger for it."

"Then there's nothing to be done?" he asked miserably.

"Oh yes, there's a great deal to be done. We must uncover that deeper fear and determine why driving triggers it. Then we can see about curing it for good."

My assurances that a cure was possible brought about an immediate reaction in George. Beginning to relax, he met my eyes with his for the first time during our session. The power of suggestion, of course, is a potent tool. Convincing a patient that help is at hand becomes an important step in aiding him to discover the root of his problem.

"George, in order to help you, I'm going to need more information than you've been able to give me . . . information that you may not even realize you possess. I'm going to use hypnosis to secure that information. You'll find that you can reach a very relaxed state by concentrating with your conscious mind on a pleasant thought. When your conscious mind is focused on that idea and very relaxed, I'll begin to probe your unconscious for the causes of this panic."

"But can it really help, doctor? I don't understand how," George protested, still skeptical.

"Yes, I'm sure it can. But let me explain by giving you an analogy. Suppose you and a friend are living in an African jungle hut. One day, as you go out for a walk, a lion suddenly leaps out at you. You're terrified. You reach for your gun, but it's not there, and that roaring lion is getting closer every second. You take to your heels in fright and race back to the hut as fast as you can with that howling beast at your back. Reaching safety in the nick of time, you slam the door behind you, shaking with fear.

"Sounds like a story with a happy ending, doesn't it? But here's the twist. Your buddy is a practical joker. While you've been chased by the roaring lion, he has recorded the terrifying experience on tape. Just when you've regained your courage and are ready to march through the door of the hut, he switches on the recording of the lion's roar. How will you react when you hear that roar?"

"Back away from the door, I guess—stay inside."

"That's right. You remain inside, trembling with fear. Most emotional distress results from the unconscious recording of a problem that hasn't been solved. With a phobia like yours, George, that recording is being triggered when you drive in the car. You're trapped by that recording just as if you were shut up in the jungle hut. We need to find a way to free you from the hut."

"How do we do that?"

"By shutting off the tape recording."

Within a few sessions I was able to determine that George's phobia was caused by two experiences in his past. As a young man he had quarreled terribly with his father, who had wanted George to settle down and find a career during a time when the son was still experiencing wanderlust. From that time on George harbored a terrible feeling of guilt for having angered his father.

The second incident, one which contributed most directly to George's driving phobia, occurred the evening before his father's funeral. George was flying to join his mother for the service when the plane was buffeted by a tremendous storm. He felt certain that he was going to be killed because he had been angry with his father. He was especially frightened because he felt that he deserved to be punished for his treatment of his father.

George was imprisoned in the cells of guilt and fear. Every time he climbed into his car, unconscious memories of his terrible plane trip were released. In his unconscious mind he was up in that plane, ready to be killed for having angered his father.

Once George and I isolated and examined his problem, a cure followed rapidly. He was able to unlock his mind from the guilt of his natural anger and find freedom when hypnoanalysis provided him with the key.

Human beings can find their minds inextricably trapped in several kinds of prisons. Effectively immobilizing the sufferer without revealing any direct connection to the outside world, they are the result of faulty functioning of the mind in its comprehension of the world. Fear is probably present in all of these prisons, but never so prominently as in the phobias.

Anxiety

Anxiety and acute anxiety attacks are another manifestation of a powerful fear imprisoning the mind. Unlike phobias, the fear is not related to any specific circumstances, although it might be just as severe. If you can imagine yourself feeling frightened or apprehensive for no obvious reason, you can appreciate the tensions which the anxiety sufferer experiences.

Edward came to see me because he had been having difficulties sleeping for over five years. He could not remember what it was like to sleep soundly throughout the night, but he had no idea what kept him awake so often. He was only able to sleep if he took a very heavy dose of a sleeping medication, but this had the predictable effect of making him quite drowsy the following day. He experimented for a time with alcohol but gave this up when he sensed the possibility of addiction.

Edward's days were also unpleasantly colored by constant feelings of tension. He suffered from headaches which usually started in the back of the neck. A constant worrier, he was always preparing himself for things to go wrong—and, of course, they frequently did. He spent much of his time fretting about things that might not happen but felt that he must be mentally prepared for any eventuality.

When he did find rest, he experienced dreadful dreams in which he was either being chased by some unnamed and unidentifiable horror or he was falling, falling, falling. As far as he could remember, he always awakened before hitting the ground.

During the day Edward felt tired and exhausted. He was seldom able to complete self-appointed tasks and frequently had to lie down to rest. He knew that he was constantly in a state of nervous tension but felt powerless to do anything about it. Edward's story has been repeated by many of my patients over the years. A physician who has been in practice for any length of time will have encountered this problem but usually has found it difficult to treat.

Chronic anxiety, another cell in the prison of fear, can ensnare the mind. Due to fear less specific than the fear associated with phobias, it is present constantly, regardless of external circumstances.

2. The Prison of Anger

Anger imprisons the mind as effectively as fear. It is a normal human emotion which administers its most crippling effect when its expression is prohibited. Anger can be repressed but never eradicated. It continues to seek release by expressing itself in an abnormal but somewhat disguised manner. We will later consider why anger is sometimes not permitted normal expression, but here we seek to understand what may happen when the normal avenues of expression are blocked.

Migraine

Migraine is a common form of headache, responsible for an enormous amount of human distress. It is an excellent example of what may happen when anger is repressed instead of granted normal expression.

Tom came to see me with a migraine problem. Apart from these headaches, he declared, he was very happy. At 40 years of age he enjoyed a lovely wife and two healthy teenage daughters. His world appeared to be perfect.

Only a migraine sufferer can really appreciate the relentless severity of an attack. Tom explained that he frequently went to bed feeling quite well, but shortly after wakening the next morning, his head would begin to throb with pain situated over the left eye. Usually the pain would increase unless his medication, always at hand, was immediately effective. If it was not, he would be incapacitated for the remainder of that day and sometimes well into the following day.

Sometimes he would reach his office and be able to work for a few hours, but then the headache would become so intense that he would find it impossible to continue. Returning home to bed, he would remain in a darkened room with appropriate doses of medication. On occasion he became so ill that he called his doctor for an injection to relieve the pain. On other occasions he would vomit, which seemed to relieve him. Usually after a good sleep, Tom would awaken feeling well, able once again to continue his normal life.

Before consulting me, Tom's headaches had become much more frequent. In the previous year they had begun to recur at approximately two-week intervals. He had tried many medications and found that although none completely prevented the attacks, he would often experience some relief from pain if he took them far enough in advance. He had undergone all the investigations that were medically recommended, but no evidence of any disease had been detected. He was regarded as healthy and physically very fit. No one knew what brought on his headaches, but they certainly caused him and his family excessive misery.

Prior to therapy I did not know the cause of Tom's headaches, but I suspected, from my previous experience with this problem, that they were probably the result of suppressed anger. Tom maintained that he never lost his temper, always keeping a tight rein upon it because he could not bear to hurt anyone's feelings. He recognized himself as a perfectionist who must always do things absolutely correctly so that no one could possibly find fault with his work.

Happily, through analytical hypnotherapy, Tom was eventually able to discover the cause of his migraine, which indeed proved to be repressed anger, and to find new means of dealing with it.

Suppressed anger is like a sleeping volcano; it can erupt periodically in the form of a headache, backache or some other physical discomfort.

Peptic Ulcer

A peptic ulcer is another psychosomatic illness which can result from repressed anger.

Alan's history exemplifies this problem well. He came to see me some time ago because he was suffering from a great deal of abdominal pain in spite of extensive surgical treatment for a stomach ulcer. Because of occasional bleeding from the operation site, further surgery had been recommended. He had come to the conclusion that repeated operations had not brought any permanent improvement in his health, so he was desperate to try an alternative form of therapy.

Alan was an engineer in his late forties who felt frustrated in a job which made few demands upon him intellectually. He found that he was frequently being called upon to do his work in a manner which he considered to be inefficient and unsatisfactory. Fancying himself more informed than his superiors, he was frequently forced to suppress his opposition to them on important issues. Often depressed and lacking in energy, he persistently looked upon himself as a personal failure.

After talking to Alan for a short time, I became aware of the tremendous potential that lay dormant in him. He had been able to use this potential by starting a small business in the sale of tools which, with the help of his wife, he operated in addition to his job as an engineer. Although quite successful, he remained dissatisfied with his efforts. He wanted to change his life in some way but did not know how. I received the impression that Alan was a man with enormous energy which somehow had been obstructed. This is the very kind of personality, of course, that is prone to suffer from psychosomatic illnesses, and we will later learn how people like Alan are imprisoned by the anger they cannot express. I am pleased to say that Alan was eventually able to escape from his prison and become virtually free of his symptoms.

Back Pain

Many people who suffer from low back pain can find no cause for its origin. Their x-rays are normal, and clinical signs do not indicate any disease; yet the pain recurs intermittently year after year.

Mary came to see me because she had heard that hypnosis could help to relieve pain. She was fed up with having to take medication for a back pain that had plagued her for over twenty years. At the time I met her, she was in her mid-forties with a grown-up family. I recall that she displayed the resigned look of extensive suffering. She was quite handsome and well-dressed with a quiet voice and demeanor which suggested someone who would prefer not to be noticed. She told me that her only periods of freedom from the back pain, which was sometimes quite excruciating, occurred during her pregnancies. This is, of course, quite unlike an organic ailment, which would tend to worsen during pregnancy. She admitted to being tense and depressed, but she attributed this to her back pain, which she felt would make anyone feel depressed. It certainly prevented her from performing a variety of tasks, and it particularly hindered her from sharing in activities with the rest of the family. Often she had to retire to bed while her husband and children went on their way without her.

Mary believed that her back pain physically imprisoned her, but in therapy she learned that her real prison was one of unexpressed anger. Once she was able to vent that anger, she freed herself from it and her back pain.

Hypertension

High blood pressure or hypertension is a very serious modern disease which appears to be on the increase. We physicians know that the strain which it imposes upon the heart and the blood vessels is

11

frequently responsible for disability and often leads to early death. Modern medical treatment is often highly effective in controlling high blood pressure but rarely succeeds in curing it. This is because only in a minority of cases can a cause be found and treated. In my experience, the origin of hypertension is usually an emotional tension which results from a blocking of the expression of anger.

Phillip was thirty-eight years of age when he first consulted me. He was overweight and suffering from high blood pressure which, without continuous medication, soared into a range which could soon lead to permanent damage to his heart, kidneys or blood vessels. He was aware that any of these eventualities could cause his death, and he was told that losing some weight would go a long way to achieving control of his blood pressure.

Although a big man, Phillip was quiet and retiring. He was always smiling and was very well liked. He would never argue with anyone and would certainly never be the cause of an argument. He had never been heard to defend himself, and it would require a great effort of imagination to think of him becoming angry. Phillip did admit to a great deal of tension and to suffering from difficulty in falling asleep. He also felt that he was totally unable to stop himself from eating fattening foods.

In therapy we found a seething anger within Phillip which was kept so totally controlled that he was entirely unaware of it. The only external evidence of the anger was his raised blood pressure and his self-destructive eating pattern. He was imprisoned by his anger, and only when he realized this was he able to do something to release it and thus to free himself from its prison. When that happened he became more relaxed, his blood pressure started to fall and he was at last able to stay on a reducing diet program.

Obesity
Because overeating may result from a variety of causes, the problem of obesity becomes exceedingly complex. One of the most common reasons for obesity is suppressed anger. Typically, the obese woman is one who always appears to be jovial and without a care in the world. She even shares in jokes about being overweight. Deep inside, however, she is boiling with anger from the hurts that she has received. Yet she continues to swallow her anger with every mouthful of food.

I well remember Peggy, who at twenty-five had attractive features, suggesting that she might have been extremely beautiful with one hundred pounds less weight. When she came to me for help, she explained that she had been only one hundred and fifteen pounds when she married at sixteen. Pregnant at the time of her first visit, and having two other children, she attributed much of her excess weight to her pregnancies, for she had lost very little after each. Her younger child was then four years of age, and she eventually admitted to putting on about fifty pounds since his birth. Like so many obese people, she found it difficult to accept responsibility for her increased weight.

Peggy told me a great deal about herself. She had few friends, but she frequently visited her mother, who lived not far from her. She seldom enjoyed these visits because her mother was extremely critical of her. She did not think that her mother intended to hurt her, but this was simply her way. Peggy felt that nothing could be done about it. Her husband worked at a distance from home and was rarely at home except on weekends. She did not like this but knew that she had to tolerate it for the time being. Peggy had never endured any financial problems, but she was often depressed for no clear reason. Finally, she had a daughter of eight who presented her with discipline problems.

During hypnoanalysis we discovered that Peggy was indeed seething with tremendous anger of which she was initially quite oblivious. An old anger which she could not let herself feel, let alone express, it was the force which drove her to eat even though she was not hungry. Only when she came to terms with her anger and accepted it did she escape from its prison. When she first came to me, she thought that she would get rid of her compulsion to eat simply by means of a posthypnotic suggestion given in hypnosis. Unfortunately, solutions are not easily available, and suggestions given in this manner are usually rejected or followed for a short time only.

Since the problem of obesity is so important, I shall be discussing it in greater depth elsewhere in this book, and we will discover that repressed anger is only one of its possible causes.

3. The Prison Of Pain and Sadness

The deep wound and the sadness of rejection is probably central to the genesis of all emotional illnesses. The earlier such rejection occurs, the more devastating its effect, for the child who has never experienced acceptance commands few resources with which to deal with later rejection. The person who plays the greatest part in the creation of a child's mental health is clearly inevitably his mother.

Her acceptance enables him to accept himself. Rejection by mother is always acutely painful and frightening.

The pain of rejection is often too severe to tolerate at a conscious level and therefore must be repressed. It does not go away, however, no matter how unaware the individual is of its existence. Its constant demand to be expressed in some form or other results in a physical or an emotional disturbance—or a combination of both. Only a few examples can be given here.

Asthma

We can verify a strong allergic element in asthma, a condition in which the victim suffers great difficulty in breathing. There is some evidence to suggest that even this element has an emotional basis, but in any case, it is generally agreed that emotion can aggravate almost any allergic illness, and this was certainly never more true than with asthma.

I first met Albert some years ago when he was referred to me because his asthma attacks appeared to be increasing in frequency. At the time he was twenty, and he informed me that he had suffered from this problem since the age of four. The younger of two boys, Albert recalled that his brother was apparently brighter than he and did very well at school, whereas he did comparatively badly. He blamed that on his asthma, which frequently kept him at home and made it difficult for him to compete with the others.

Some of Albert's asthma attacks had been frighteningly severe, and he had been hospitalized on occasions to the great disruption of the family. His parents appeared to be quite devoted to him, and he felt that he related well to them.

Strangely enough, Albert was free of all attacks of asthma for one year. During this year he was away from home attending college in another city. In the eighteen months or so following his return from college, his attacks increased in severity. Medications had to be increased, and he was eventually placed on cortisone therapy, which gave him some relief from the intensity of the attacks but did not reduce their frequency. He came to see me specifically to help him reduce his attacks of asthma so that he could discontinue some of his medications.

During analysis we discovered that the true cause of his asthma was his intense feeling of rejection. His asthma represented a silent cry of pain, expressing a hurt which he could not allow himself to feel. It was necessary for Albert to deal with his pain before his asthma eventually improved.

Depression
Each of us has experienced a fit of melancholy, but depression possesses a certain futile and groundless quality which sets it apart from ordinary sadness. Typically the sufferer is unable to function properly. He becomes easily tired and does not sleep well. He is irritable and frequently unaccountably tearful. During periods of depression the world appears an awful and hopeless place in which nothing ever goes right. Depression is often complicated by feelings of anger and guilt, both of which can be traced to experiences of early rejection. The rejection is responsible for the sadness and the anger, but this anger may be repressed or directed toward the sufferer. Alternatively, the sadness may be concealed by the anger, and neither the sadness nor the anger will be given appropriate external expression. For this reason the depressed person may express his anger against himself in the extremely hostile act of suicide—the murder of the self.

Sandra was a tall, attractive girl in her late twenties who had lived with several men but had never married. She was sustaining a relationship with a married man who was separated from his wife at the time that she consulted me. Her history was an emotionally stormy one. There had been many admissions to a hospital for psychiatric treatment during her adolescence, on one occasion she attempted suicide by slashing her wrists and on another by taking an overdose of tranquilizers.

She came to see me because, once again feeling depressed and hopeless, she was searching for a different route to the solution of her emotional problems. She was aware of her sadness but was unaware of its true intensity or of the anger which accompanied it. I suspected that she would have difficulty in coming to terms with the immense amount of repressed hurt that needed to be dealt with, and so it proved. She did, however, eventually succeed in dealing with the pain and sadness which was imprisoning her in a life of self-rejection, and she was ultimately able to gain the freedom of self-acceptance. This has resulted in many changes in her life and in her relationships. She now possesses an understanding of her former behavior and knows that it has ended for good.

Depression is a clear sign of rejection, originally parental, which manifests itself in the form of self-rejection. Feelings of rejection appear so commonly in analysis that I deem them to be ever present in emotional disturbances.

Drug Addiction

Society has always relied heavily on drugs. Even primitive man learned that certain herbs could modify the feelings in his body and mind. Man has regularly turned to medicines of different kinds to help heal sickness, and as a general physician in family practice I must have prescribed many thousands of dollars' worth of drugs over the years.

It is therefore not surprising that some of us come to rely so heavily on a particular drug for its effectiveness in relieving a specific discomfort, that we cannot give it up. Drug addiction is a serious problem since its side effects frequently create a situation far worse than that they were intended to relieve. Alcohol, tobacco, tranquilizers, amphetamines and heroin are but a few of the drugs whose addictive properties have created worldwide problems. There is little evidence that the many legal restraints have been successful in modifying drug addiction in any way.

An understanding of the reasons for drug addiction makes it clear why legal restraints are doomed to failure. All drugs are taken voluntarily only if they succeed in relieving a discomfort and/or giving a pleasurable feeling. I believe that those who become addicted to a drug are suffering from a severe pain which is largely or entirely unconscious. The pain is always intense but is consciously only felt as an uneasiness, clamoring to be soothed. The drug is therefore being used by the addict to suppress this severe unconscious pain, though its success is only temporary. Furthermore, the effectiveness of the drug frequently decreases so that additional doses, with a concomitant increase in side effects, become necessary for effective control of the unconscious pain. However, when unconscious pain requires relief, the thought of future discomfort from the side effects of the drug is rarely an effective deterrent to its use. This is particularly the case if such pain is more severe than the side effects of the drug or the legal deterrents.

Alcoholism

Alcoholism is the most common example of drug addiction. Probably every one of us knows, or has known, an alcoholic and has wondered why he continues to treat himself in this self-destructive manner.

John was referred to me because of his smoking habit but confided that he really wanted help with his alcohol problem. A big man both physically and mentally, John has done very well in his occupation, and when I first saw him, he had reached a very important executive position in his firm. He was then about forty-five years of age and had everything that one could wish for—a lovely wife, three children who were all doing well at school and college, a house, a cottage, and many other joys of life which should have made him feel secure and happy. Yet he confided that every so often he would become very depressed and would embark upon an alcoholic binge which would prevent him from functioning for several days. Recognizing his illness but incapable of identifying its origin, he was seeking my help to assist him in controlling the habit.

I guessed from my previous experience with alcoholics that John was nursing a deep distress which periodically surfaced but which he was unable to feel, recognize or face. This indeed proved to be the case. When John came to terms with a great deal of hidden pain, he was eventually able to relinquish it permanently. His problems with alcohol since then have faded because without pain, he no longer needs the pain killer alcohol.

Excessive Smoking

A high proportion of heavy smokers can be persuaded to give up smoking by direct suggestion in hypnosis, but a significant number cannot. These people rely upon cigarettes to ease unconscious pain and distress. Only when that pain is resolved by the application of mature understanding to the attendant problem can the tension creating the compulsion to smoke be relieved and the direct suggestion to give up smoking be accepted. So it is with all drug addictions. The pain must be dealt with before the habit can be permanently relinquished.

The success rate for hypnotherapy in helping people to quit smoking or to give up any other addiction must always be less than satisfactory until they can be released from their prison of unconscious pain.

4. The Prison Of Guilt

In order to make comprehensible my concept of emotional illness, I have artificially separated the three prisons of fear, anger and hurt, but I believe that all of these, in effect, are adjacent to and overlap each other with intercommunicating doors, so that any or all of these emotions might be involved in the production of illness from mental imprisonment.

I come now to the fourth prison, that of guilt, which is always closely connected to the first three. We shall discover how guilt is consistently a potent factor in the production of all emotional illnesses. Under certain conditions the feeling of guilt plays a prominent part in the emotional problem.

Impotence

In no other condition is guilt more likely to be the main causative factor in the production of symptoms than in the condition of impotence, the failure of the male to perform satisfactorily during sexual intercourse. It has been acknowledged more and more as a cause of considerable unhappiness for many married couples and, in these days of greater acceptance of extra-marital sex, has been viewed as a source of problems in these relationships also.

Today many therapies directed at resolving this problem are meeting with varying degrees of success. However, persistent unconscious feelings of guilt will continue to prevent success in a significant proportion of cases.

Edwin was referred to me because at the age of forty-five he had found himself to be impotent. He did experience penile erections from time to time, but he was unable to maintain an erection long enough to have satisfactory intercourse. He had been a widower for five years. His wife had died from cancer, and he had nursed her during the illness. Theirs had been a love match, and sex with her, though infrequent, had always been very good until her illness, when he had naturally ceased making any sexual demands upon her. Terribly depressed by his wife's death, a long time had elapsed before he had been able to socialize again. Reacquaintance with an old girlfriend developed a relationship which they decided to cement by marriage. With that commitment they began a sexual relationship, but Edwin discovered to his dismay and embarrassment that he was impotent.

Edwin's doctor administered medication, injections and advice to no avail, and Edwin was doubtful whether he should go ahead with his plans for remarriage. He had even begun to wonder whether he had become too old to start a new sexual relationship.

I knew that this was not true, and I also guessed that his problem was too deep to be resolved merely by direct suggestion in hypnosis, which is often quite effective. In fact, his case required some thorough investigation, using analytical hypnotic techniques, before we were able to locate and deal with the cause of his problem. It was, of course, a strong feeling of guilt about this new relationship which he was totally unaware of at a conscious level. After we were able to relieve the guilt feeling, Edwin was able to function quite normally in his sexual relationship. He is now happily married.

Frigidity

This is the female equivalent of impotence in the male, and although sexual problems in the female are probably just as common as in the male, they are less often the presenting problem for which therapy is sought. It is possible for the female to function sexually even though she is emotionally detached or even opposed to sex. Usually, this problem comes to light as part of a wider emotional disturbance which is disrupting her life.

Angela was about thirty years of age when she consulted me because of her recurrent depressions. She had been married for more than ten years, but throughout that time she had never really enjoyed her sexual life with her husband. She recalled that their premarital sex had been quite good.

During therapy for her depression we uncovered an enormous amount of guilt associated with sex, and it was clear that she had blocked off her sexual feelings because of her guilt regarding them. We also needed to understand why this guilt did not prevent her from enjoying her premarital sex. With this full understanding she was eventually able to relinquish all of her guilt feelings. She not only stopped being depressed but also once again allowed herself to enjoy sex with her husband.

Any woman who is suffering from an inability to enjoy normal sexual feelings is probably suffering from guilt, and to this extent she is imprisoned by it.

Obesity

We have already spoken about the problem of obesity, but I mention it again here because it is sometimes a manifestation of imprisonment in the prison of guilt. In such cases the sufferer is the victim of a compulsion to eat, even when he is not aware of any desire to eat. The compulsion, which is self-punishing, results from an intense unconscious feeling of guilt.

Twenty-two-year-old Rosalyn provides a striking history of someone who becomes a victim of this compulsion. She requested that I give her a posthypnotic suggestion not to eat because she was aware that she was eating unconsciously. She would go for days on an excellent diet program and then, for no apparent reason, would become obsessed by the urge to eat. Stopping at the local store, she would buy all kinds of junk foods, take them home and gorge herself on them, stuffing food into herself until she could hardly move. These were labeled "binges," and she was deeply ashamed of her failure to control them. Not consciously aware of any problem that could trigger her gormandizing, she agreed to analytical hypnotherapy.

Rosalyn was quite surprised when we located an experience which she recalled consciously but did not at all associate with intense feelings of guilt. The association had been suppressed. Only after she became aware of her guilt feelings and the reasons for them was Rosalyn able to dismiss them. When she was freed from her prison of guilt, she successfully maintained her reducing diet and consistently lost weight.

When imprisoned by guilt, the victim can only alleviate that guilt by some assault upon himself. Overeating is one common means of self-aggression, but there are many others.

Skin Diseases

It has long been known that skin diseases are strongly affected by emotional factors. In fact, many of them are due to unconscious feelings of guilt. This may at first sound far-fetched, but the improvement of several patients has been the direct result of relinquishing such guilt feelings.

I remember the case of Martha, who at forty-five years of age had suffered from urticaria, popularly known as hives, for many years. It frequently involves the mucous membranes as well as the skin. She experienced these attacks at odd times, and the search for an allergic cause proved to be unfruitful. Occasionally she became so swelled up with urticaria attacks involving mouth and throat that her breathing was threatened and emergency treatment had to be adopted. Following therapy, during which she was able to deal with an apparently unrelated source of guilt, her urticaria stopped recurring and she has remained free from it ever since.

Suicide

We cannot leave a discussion of the prison of guilt without taking a brief look at the problem of suicide, which I shall explore in greater detail later.

Why should anyone wish to kill himself? Those who have themselves attempted suicide may understand its causes to a certain extent, but it is my experience that the reasons for suicide are only dimly understood, even by those who are deeply involved in working with the problem.

Sometimes the victim has been known to undergo a prolonged period of depression, but often there has been no prior warning. The individual may even have appeared to be the life and soul of the party. He was perhaps occasionally a little moody, but on the whole he seemed to enjoy life.

Suicide is the ultimate hostile act. It is the murder of oneself, and yet for the perpetrator it seems to be the right and proper act to perform at the time. He feels that he is killing a monster who has no right to live and is thereby doing the world a favor. In fact, he declares that this may be the only positive feat he has ever performed. This sounds like absurd thinking to the observer, but one has to be inside the victim's mind to recognize his logic. From his perspective he has no alternative; only because we cannot penetrate his rationale do we fail to understand him.

He is living in a prison of guilt, certain that he can only escape through death. Furthermore, he is sure that this is an appropriate gesture because he unconsciously believes that he has been sentenced to death and this is only carrying out that sentence. We shall analyze this viewpoint in greater detail later, attempting to understand the suicide's thinking at an unconscious level. Many of us living in prisons of guilt are potential suicides but are using various methods to ward off the death sentence.

Jennifer came to see me because she was entertaining frightening thoughts that she should kill herself. At twenty-four years of age, she had recently graduated from the university and was apparently doing quite well in her chosen profession as a social worker. She described her recent states of depression and complained that she found it difficult to concentrate upon her work. She had good reason to seek help from these suicidal feelings because some ten years or so before she had made an almost successful attempt to take her own life. She was only saved by prompt and efficient medical treatment.

Having heard of the facility with which hypnosis could uncover unconscious thought, Jennifer hoped that I could help. We found, as I expected we might, that she had always been in a prison of guilt and had existed with a sentence of death hanging over her head since birth. It had never been commuted but only postponed to the end of her university training. Her case was very complex, but we were eventually able to reach a resolution which enabled her to escape from the prison of guilt to a freedom she had never previously known.

In discussing the main prisons of the mind, I have only mentioned a few of the many problems which are presented to hypnotherapists each day. In almost every case I am able to find some evidence of emotional incarceration in one or more of the four prisons that I have described.

No one chooses to go to prison, so when I discover a patient tucked away in one of these prisons, I naturally ask, How did he get there? What crime did he commit which led to his prison sentence? And what is his sentence?

By seeking and finding answers to questions such as these, I am able to help the victim determine the means of securing a release from his prison. However, before we get to that point, I want to discuss the crimes which are present in the emotional code—very different from offenses listed in the criminal code of any modern society, but nonetheless capable of landing one in solitary confinement.

Chapter Two

The crime

In the eyes of the law, a crime is any act that endangers the peace and order of society. To maintain its good health societies must apprehend and punish those who defy its rules. Criminals must not be allowed to repeat their offenses.

I intend to draw a close parallel between this generally accepted understanding of crime and the crime which results in the imprisonment of part of our minds. This latter crime differs from the usual crime only in that the society involved is an extremely small one. It usually consists of the individual and one other person, most often mother.

Seen from outside the small society of the persons involved these acts do not appear to be crimes. Even the individuals involved have difficulty in recognizing these events as crimes when they viewed them from the distance that time eventually imposes.

I am here

As I became more involved in analytical hypnotherapy I discovered that a high proportion of my patients' problems appeared to begin at birth or even before. Initially, I had some difficulty in fully accepting this startling discovery. Other workers in hypnotherapy have come to similar conclusions in recent years. There now seems to be little doubt that the circumstances of birth and sometimes of pregnancy can provide us with solutions to emotional problems which previously appeared insoluble.

As a result of this finding, which is so important to analytical hypnotherapy as to be almost revolutionary, I now routinely employ techniques which enable my patients to explore these early experiences. In this manner we are able to discover whether any circumstances associated with birth might have been responsible for an emotional problem.

I once believed that the unborn child and newborn infant could not be aware of any of the events occurring so early in life. I now have abundant and irrefutable evidence that I was wrong. True, consciousness does not develop until the early years of childhood, but I now know that the unconscious mind is highly developed in the prenatal period. Indeed, it is sufficiently developed to be able to record accurately all significant events occurring at that time. These events, which may have a profound effect on the remainder of the individual's life, require to be fully understood if the resulting problems are to be resolved.

Emotional problems can commence in the prenatal period. Many patients, for instance, have taken me to this period in which the unconscious mind of the unborn baby has recorded a strong impression of rejection. He is an unwelcome burden. Perhaps the baby is not able to fully appreciate the significance of the events at the time, but I do believe that they are faithfully recorded by the unconscious mind at the moment of occurrence. They are later understood and interpreted at an unconscious level in the light of subsequent events.

The earliest crime that an individual can commit is the crime of existing. He is unwanted and therefore should not be. We have already defined a crime as an act which is a danger to the peace and order of society. An unwanted infant has clearly committed such a crime, for his very presence disturbs the existing order and peace.

Time after time I have found that feelings of guilt have originated in prenatal rejection when the unborn baby hears, or in some other way senses, that he is not welcome. Unaware that the responsibility for existence cannot be charged to the infant, he can only discern that his presence is causing distress to others and that his very existence is meeting with grave disapproval.

He has committed a crime for which he feels intense guilt. The only way in which he can expiate his crime is by not existing. It may be a long time before he learns how to accomplish this by killing himself, but before that he will discover that the compromise of being as insignificant as possible may be acceptable.

Many of my patients vaguely sense that they do not belong or that they are worthless and should not be here. They harbor insecurities which intimate that they do not deserve to be alive. This feeling pervades every thought and action so that they are unable to enjoy life. Time and again my analysis has verified that they were subjected to a strong early rejection, either before or at birth, which made them certain that they had committed the crime of being here. How often have we heard people say, "I wish I had never been born?" Some of these people have wished this from the moment of birth.

Let me tell you about Ruth. She was thirty-eight years old when she came to see me. Quietly dressed and quietly spoken, she almost appeared to melt into the background. I had the distinct impression

24

that she could not bear to be looked at or noticed, and it took a long while before we could establish a rapport. She recounted several liaisons with unsuitable men, but she had never been married. I gathered that she seldom made a success of any project that she had started. Things always seemed to go wrong for her. She had been admitted to several hospitals for the treatment of a depression which was her constant companion.

She looked quite dejected at our first meeting, and when we talked about her experiences, it seemed clear that she had succeeded in functioning only marginally throughout her life. She admitted to strong feelings of worthlessness, to the sensation that life held nothing for her. She could not make friends easily and described herself as a loner. On the other hand, she made no enemies because she was always so careful to avoid giving offense. I received a strong impression of emptiness as I counseled with her, but I found it difficult to communicate with her because she rejected the possibility that anyone could be interested in her or her problems for more than a few minutes at a time. She amply demonstrated her lack of self-esteem by the repeated question, "What good am I to anyone?" I knew that therapy in such a case would be very difficult, even though her very presence in my office reflected her personal admission that she should not continue in her present quandary.

As part of the initial analysis I regressed her to the moments immediately after birth, asking her to recall whether or not she felt welcome at that time. She indicated that she not only felt totally unwelcome but harbored guilt for being there. When I regressed her to the time that she first felt unwelcome she reverted to a moment shortly before birth. With a little encouragement she was able to recall the experience responsible for her feeling of rejection. She recollected her mother saying quite vehemently to her father, "I never wanted this baby!" Her pain in remembering the incident was very real. Feeling responsible for her mother's distress, she knew that she had committed a grave crime.

Having perpetrated the crime of existing, Ruth had been condemned to the prison of guilt. The locks were secure and well-guarded. It took a great deal of ingenuity to free her, to persuade her to accept the right to live. It may yet be some time before she can fully accept her freedom.

This particular crime, the crime of existing, has received little attention from psychiatrists since it is only readily recognizable by the employment of hypnoanalytical techniques. Its importance in the etiology of mental illness, however, cannot be overestimated. A knowledge of the existence of this crime frequently gives a much clearer understanding of an emotional problem.

I am a girl/boy

During hypnoanalysis we often discover that feelings of rejection are rooted in the patient's belief that he or she is of the wrong sex. The guilt can be just as traumatic as that discussed above. Because the newborn is not aware that his sex is anyone's responsibility but his own, he feels a personal liability for the distress that his sex has brought to his parent. He feels rejected at a time when acceptance is crucial. If the infant is a boy when the parents desired a girl, he will try earnestly to behave as a girl in order to receive acceptance. Success in this venture, of course, will be very limited apart from those exceptional cases in which this guilt can at last be expiated later in life by a sex change operation. I believe that in many cases homosexuality can be traced to this crime. Certainly all transvestism is rooted here.

Lesley came to me at the age of nineteen for help in losing weight. Early in hypnoanalysis she recalled her father's intense disappointment shortly after her birth when he learned that she was a girl. Because it was important to her that she be accepted by him, she was crushed by his rejection of her female identity. Other later experiences reinforced her guilt about not being a boy. Throughout her life she had desperately tried to make amends for the "crime" by behaving as much like a boy as possible.

Lesley recalled that she often wore male clothing and played hockey and football with the boys. She seemed to despise girls and felt compelled to compete with boys. She became very depressed at puberty when she began to menstruate and her breasts started to develop, for she knew then that she could never really please her father and that he would not accept what she could no longer deny— that she was a girl! At this time she sought solace in food, which she later recognized as another way of denying her femininity. Only when Lesley could learn to accept herself as a girl was she able to control her eating and lose weight. Released from her prison of guilt, she could view herself as a unique individual.

Lesley's story is being repeated almost daily in my office. Sexual difficulties are naturally quite common with these people. Their guilt about their own sex prevents them from functioning adequately as sexual beings. Feelings of unworthiness and depression are natural responses to rejection, and obesity is a common way for women to deny their femininity.

26

I am angry

Just as gender can create rejection, certain human traits may occasion distress, causing the individual to feel that he has committed a crime. Every human being possesses emotions, which are his unconscious means of responding to the world around him and form an essential part of his survival mechanism.

The crime of being angry is perpetrated with regularity because it is one of the primary emotions which function to protect us. It is present in all human beings and most animals. Uncontrolled anger, however, produces alarming consequences, and all societies exert some control over it. Some regard anger as so abhorrent that its expression is emphatically deplored.

In conducting hypnoanalysis, I often determine that the world of the infant or child has been jolted by parental injustice. As a result, the child is frustrated and becomes angry. If the parent's responses are extreme, the patient may be severely reprimanded and subjected to a frightening display of anger, and thus the infant or child will quickly become aware that he has committed a crime. He feels angry but discovers that he must not express that anger. Only bad people are angry.

A small child does not understand bad or good. However, he readily comprehends parental acceptance and rejection. We shall later see how the idea of "being bad" is associated with parental rejection. Since every child needs parental acceptance because of the protection and security that it engenders, he will repress his normal anger in order to gain it.

We have already seen that anger can be repressed but never abolished. The child who has been convicted of the crime of anger learns that he must not even allow himself to feel that emotion, and thus becomes locked in a prison of anger.

Phyllis came to see me because she had heard that hypnosis was often useful in helping people lose weight. She was about fifty years of age when we met, a pleasant person with a gentle air. As it turned out, she was a deeply religious woman who wished to generate only kind thoughts and perform only kind deeds. Phyllis contemplated hypnosis in desperation, uncertain whether it was the work of God or the Devil. Eventually assured that God had sent her to me, she was able to speak freely about her problem. She was seventy pounds overweight, and the fact that she was unable to diet for more than a few days at a time filled her with great shame.

Her husband, she informed me, frightened her with his outbursts of temper. He often treated her with ridicule and contempt, but she bore these assaults on her feelings with saint-like tolerance. She wondered, however, why she so often felt impelled to eat after one of these outbursts. I guessed at the reason immediately but awaited the outcome of hypnoanalysis to verify my suspicions.

In hypnoanalysis we soon located the origin of her problem. She was five years of age when her three-year-old sister wanted to take away a toy that she was playing with. As she scuffled with her sister over the toy, it caught her sister just above the eye, lacerating it severely. Her sister screamed, her mother screamed, and even her father, normally very calm and impartial, yelled at her. She was terrified. Banished to her room while her sister was rushed to hospital under the impending threat of blindness, Phyllis immediately recognized that she had committed the grevious crime of anger.

At that point Phyllis realized that she must never be angry again. Others might be permitted an outburst of anger, but not Phyllis. She was a bad girl who must not even feel anger, let alone express it. Her guilt locked her firmly in the prison of anger, but her anger never really left her. We learned that her husband frequently made her feel very angry, yet she was never consciously aware of it. Resentment was consistently sublimated and controlled by food.

It took some time for Phyllis to realize that she was no more responsible for her sister's accident than her sister was herself. She also had to learn that her anger was not really bad, that she had a right to protect herself against her husband's unfair attacks. When she was able to understand this, she accepted her anger, remembering that Christ had also vented His anger at the appropriate time. As a result, she was freed from her prison of anger and was at last able to adhere to a diet program.

I am afraid

We are all prone to fear. It is an important protective emotion which not only warns us of danger but also mobilizes our flight responses so that we can flee from peril.

Sometimes an intensely frightening experience has occurred, but for some reason the natural response of fear is unacceptable or meets with marked parental disapproval, preventing its full expression. During these circumstances the frightened child feels that he has committed a crime. He is afraid, but because his fear is unacceptable, he must lock it up and become incarcerated within his prison of fear, from which he cannot escape in lieu of parental disapproval and the guilt that this involves.

Since it is very easy to commit this crime, many of my patients turn out to be hardened criminals. I recall a young man of about thirty years of age who came to me for help with a stammer. As far as George knew, he had always stammered quite badly. He clearly knew what he wanted to say, but he would get stuck on certain words, uttering them only after a long struggle or devising an alternative word. At times he spoke without any trace of an impediment, but at other times his speech pattern would cause great discomfort to the listener.

George particularly stressed that he had great difficulty talking in a group or addressing anyone whom he felt was his superior. He primarily stammered in new situations and among strangers. He had no difficulty in reading aloud when he was by himself. His handicap, which caused him a great deal of embarrassment, had defied all treatment by speech therapists.

In hypnoanalysis we discovered the cause of his stammering. At the age of five he was awakened from his sleep by a terrible commotion. His drunken father was storming at his mother, who was crying and screaming for his father to leave her alone. When George hurried downstairs to investigate, he saw his father preparing to strike his mother. Rushing between them in an attempt to stop his father, he was thrown to the ground; subsequently he picked himself up and hid behind the settee. As the fight grew in intensity, George was terrified. There was a sudden climax to the noise and commotion, at which point his mother's voice ceased. He was seized with an even greater panic. Had his father killed her? He wanted to scream, but he did not dare. When his father went out a few moments later, George emerged from his hiding place to find his mother conscious but dazed and bleeding from a head wound. He tried to administer comfort, but he was so frightened that he could not speak. He had stammered ever since.

George's speech impediment was corrected only after he escaped from the prison of repressed fear. When he recognized what had been obstructing his natural expression of fear, the physical defect faded.

I hurt

Our most fundamental emotion involves an awareness of pain. The trauma of rejection, whether imagined or real, is the most severe. We seldom convey this hurt in a comprehensible manner, and so its clumsy expression is met with a stern admonishment. The message becomes clear. Hurting is wrong. Feeling pain is a crime. Unfortunately, the more we try not to feel hurt, the more our discomfort grows.

At twenty-three years of age Sarah was an attractive woman who had struggled through an adventure-filled and stormy life. She came to see me because of her addiction to certain drugs. Although she had received some psychiatric treatment for this and for depression, three fairly serious suicide attempts had driven her to seek further counsel.

When I met her, she was divorced, had two children and was living with a man with a long criminal record. She herself had been a juvenile offender and was sequestered in detention homes for lengthy periods. In a flat and casual tone she informed me that she did not care about anyone or anything, including herself. As an afterthought she excluded her children from this. She appeared to despise any display of emotion and certainly showed none.

Therapy with her was long and difficult, for it embraced many traumatic episodes. The earliest of these occurred when she was about eighteen months of age. Awakened suddenly by a sharp pain between her legs, she suddenly realized that her brother was attacking her sexually. She screamed out in terror and pain. Her brother fled, but she continued to scream. A short time later her father rushed into the room. Since she was too upset to be coherent, he yelled at her for waking him up. He slapped her cruelly and warned that he would "beat the daylights out of her" if she wasn't quiet. She quickly became very quiet—and she is still quiet. Although unconsciously she knew that her hurt continued, she was unable to admit it. In her eyes the open avowal of pain was a serious crime, and she could not admit that to anyone, not even to herself. Much of her subsequent behavior was understandable as a means adopted to relieve this unconscious hurt. Drugs serve as an effective but temporary vehicle for doing this.

The crime of hurting is very common—so common, indeed, that I tend to look for it whenever I hear a patient say that he "does not care." This phrase is a strong clue that he is locked in a prison of pain for the crime of hurting.

I love

Loving is a normal human feeling. We love those with whom we feel a close bond, people who help us to feel good about ourselves and with whom we feel at ease. Being with them gives us pleasure. Whenever love is misunderstood, the insecure observer may regard it as a threat worthy only of his extreme disapproval. In such circum-

30

stances loving may be viewed as wrong, a crime as serious as the disapproval it engenders. An individual who has been accused of the crime of loving may be unable to deny it, but he can prevent it happening again.

Jennifer was a very beautiful twenty-three-year-old girl who came to me because of her difficulties with sex. She is married and has one child, but she rarely experienced any pleasure from sex. In fact, she was unable to achieve an orgasm during intercourse with her husband.

Jennifer felt that her life was incomplete. She admitted to having been somewhat promiscuous prior to her marriage and unfaithful during it, but her husband was totally unaware of this. Yet she felt very guilty about her lapses and tried to make amends by being an extremely efficient housewife. Much of the time she felt depressed and restless. She was irritable with her four-year-old son, a quiet and inoffensive child who, she knew, could not be held responsible for her feelings of frustration. She was also frequently ill-tempered with her long-suffering husband and picked quarrels with him for no good reason.

In hypnoanalysis Jennifer was able to locate an important experience which occurred when she was about the age of six. Her father, whom she loved very much, was sick in bed. She had just come home from school and decided to hurry up to his bedroom for a visit. Her father was sitting up in bed when she entered the bedroom. Since she loved her daddy so much, she took the opportunity to climb into bed and snuggle up to him. Within a short period of time her mother came home and found the two in bed together. Angry and distraught, her mother screamed, "Get the hell out of there! Don't you ever let me find you in there again!" Sobbing, Jennifer scooted out of bed and fled the room. For a long time after that she could hear her parents screaming at each other, and she was terrified at the commotion that she had caused. She had committed a terrible crime. She loved her daddy, but that had angered her mother and got her daddy into trouble. She was now certain that loving daddy was wrong, even though she could not help it. She was a criminal and must hide her crime—her love.

Jennifer did not know at that time that her father was a sexually troubled man and that her mother was only trying to protect her. Jennifer's father had made advances to her older sister, and her mother was afraid that he would attempt to molest Jennifer as well. Without an understanding of these sorry circumstances, she could only conclude that her love was a serious crime.

It soon became clear to Jennifer that she had unconsciously

31

locked up her love, but after further therapy she was able to free herself and began to love without constraint or guilt.

I am happy

Being happy is a special human experience. However, it can sometimes create problems. Happiness is frequently so rapidly and regularly followed by calamity that it would appear wiser to avoid happy experiences. Life is at least safe as long as it remains dull and prosaic.

Some of my patients have unconsciously come to the conclusion that happiness is a crime which they must avoid. Vera was one of these. She actually sought hypnotherapy to get help in losing weight. She was thirty-five but, because of an extra fifty pounds, looked much older. She had always attributed her tendency toward overweight to the fact that she could not remain on a diet long enough to reach her ideal weight. As soon as she had shed a few pounds, she would begin to feel anxious and tense; only eating some of the forbidden foods would relieve her anxiety.

Upon further discussion we found that throughout her life she had started projects full of enthusiasm, only to give them up after a while when things seemed to be going well. She was never able to reach any goals that she had set herself. Propagating feelings of uselessness and stupidity, she was genuinely surprised at her relative success in having raised three healthy and bright children. However, she worried about them a great deal and was easily depressed if anything was wrong with any of them. Her sex life was unsatisfactory, but she would not complain about that since her husband made few demands upon her sexually. She summed up her life as tedious and uninteresting. "If only I could lose some weight, perhaps things would be different," she sighed. I was certain, however, that her problem was more than fat deep.

In hypnoanalysis she took me with her to a sunny, pleasant day when she was two and a half years old. Her mother had let her out to play in the back yard, where she was having fun on the rocking horse, when the next door neighbor's lovely big dog poked his nose through the bars of the gate. She hurried over to talk to him and stroke him, but after a few moments of this Rover decided to go for a walk. Being adventurous, Vera forgot that her mummy had warned her to stay in the garden. She managed to squeeze through the bars of the gate and followed Rover along a footpath. She recalled that it was a hot day and that she had difficulty keeping up with the dog. When he eventually reached the water and went in for a swim, Vera found the water so appealing that she followed him in.

Just then Vera heard her mother's panic-stricken voice screaming, "Vera! Vera! come here at once!" She turned to greet her mother with a big, happy smile, but her mother was clearly very upset. She looked angry and frightened. Mother exclaimed, "You are a very, very bad girl! You must never do that again." Vera was not sure what she must not do again or why she was bad—or even what "bad" meant. Whatever it was, it upset mummy a great deal. Her mother threatened, "Vera, if you ever do that again, I will lock you up in the cupboard." At this Vera became frightened and sobbed violently because she recalled the terror of finding herself accidentally locked among the silent hanging clothes in pitch darkness. No, she decided right there, she would never do that again! Being happy was a crime that she must never repeat. She could not risk the terror of that cupboard! Vera had solved her problem by locking herself in an almost equally terrible place where happiness was forbidden.

She was eventually able to free herself from this prison of guilt and let herself be happy. At the same time she found that she could lose weight and that such an activity was permissible.

I am curious

At first sight it would appear that the desire to know is innocent enough and could never be construed as a crime. How can it be wrong to desire information about things that are happening in the world around us? Can this really be a crime? Yes, and we are made aware of it in the same way that we identify other crimes—by the disapproval of those to whose society we are striving to belong, namely, our parents.

Several problems led Laura to seek my help. First of all, she felt herself quite inhibited sexually and was unable to relax during intercourse. She was overweight and ate compulsively. Often very depressed, she never felt good about herself. She was aware that all of these problems were putting an almost intolerable strain upon her marriage. She was plagued by persistent feelings of worthlessness which contradicted her intellectual assessment of herself as a competent and useful human being. Suspecting an unconscious reason for her feelings, she wanted me to help her to find it. With Laura I had a feeling that I was preaching to the converted and that therapy would proceed without difficulty—and so it proved.

Laura located a critical experience which occurred when she was three years of age. Playing in the bedroom with her dolls, she heard Daddy come home. She loved her daddy very much and knew that in a little while she would get her usual big hug and a kiss. When he did not immediately come to her, she decided to go and look for him. He was not in the hall, so when she heard sounds coming from the bathroom, she decided that he must be there. Opening the bathroom door with a bang, she called, "Daddy, daddy!" Suddenly she stopped in her tracks. Daddy was there, standing in front of the toilet, holding a tube-like thing in his hand . . . and wonders upon wonders, there was water coming out of it, making a lovely noise. Laura had never seen anything so remarkable before. She gazed spellbound with such consuming interest that she did not hear Daddy telling her to get out. In fact, he was yelling, "Get the hell out of here! Mary, come and get this bloody kid out of here." Laura was so confused that she just stood there until she was hauled unceremoniously through the bathroom door by her mother.

Laura began to scream as her mother hit her repeatedly, and, it seemed, incessantly, taking no notice of Laura's cries. Why was she hitting her so? Would she never stop? Her mother screamed, "If you ever do that again, I will kill you!" and with that she threw Laura onto the bed.

Afterwards the puzzled little girl tried to discover what crime had upset Mummy and Daddy so terribly. Perhaps she loved Daddy too much. Maybe that was wrong. More than likely, however, she had found out what Daddy did in the bathroom and her mother did not want her to know. She must not be curious, for that was her crime.

Laura now understands why she had felt so guilty about sex and could not involve herself in it. She could not let herself know about such things. Eventually she was able to gain an absolute pardon for being curious and became free to enjoy a sexual relationship.

In discussing the most common crimes that human beings commit, I may have given the impression that they arise singly. Actually, the parental disapproval by which these crimes are recognized may be sufficiently strong to cause a hapless child to commit several, whether together or sequentially.

Of the crimes I have mentioned, the most serious is that of existing. Anyone who is accused of committing this crime is trapped because he continues to be a criminal every day of his life. The very process of living becomes a constant reminder of his guilt.

In the foregoing cases I have only referred to the crime which needed to be recognized before satisfactory therapy could begin. At times we discovered other crimes which had to be understood before therapy was satisfactorily concluded.

All of these crimes are really normal human attributes and activities, but the individuals accused of them are unaware of this at the time of the accusation. They are made to feel abnormal and are forced to shoulder direct responsibility for the distress caused to the parent.

Chapter Three

The Court

All societies devise a system for administering justice so that when an individual is accused of a crime, he can be tried and, if found guilty, appropriately sentenced to a designated punishment. This usually takes place in a court of law where three essential participants can be identified: the accused, the prosecutor and the judge.

The accused, or the defendant, may engage a knowledgeable associate to help him, the defense lawyer. In addition, both the defense and the prosecution may solicit witnesses to support their respective cases. These are presented in a predetermined sequence before the judge, who will decide whether the accused is guilty and what the appropriate punishment should be.

In most civilized societies this process may take considerable time in preparation and presentation before a verdict is reached. We shall see, however, that the court of the mind works much more quickly in processing all the available information and reaching a verdict— sometimes only a few seconds, and rarely more than a few days.

The mind might be compared to a highly complex computer, able to receive evidence for or against any particular course of action in order to weigh one against the other. It then makes a decision favoring one or the other according to the evidence. When an individual is accused of an emotional crime, his mind makes a decision in what I prefer to call the court of the mind. Such a decision is binding and will determine that individual's future.

The Court of the Mind

Before we can examine what happens during the trial of the accused, we need to recognize the members of the court. We can identify the accused, but who is the prosecutor? Who serves as judge? We have already specified the potential crimes and the appropriate prisons should the accused be found guilty. We need now to understand the nature and the function of each participant in the court of the mind. In order to answer some of the inevitable questions, I have turned to Eric Berne and his theories of Transactional Analysis, which have received wide support from psychotherapists in recent years.

Perhaps the greatest contribution that Eric Berne made to the understanding of human behavior was his recognition that we all function from more than one ego state. An ego state is a distinct set of feelings and behavior patterns. Each of us has at least three ego states, three different viewpoints. These ego states, labeled Child, Parent and Adult, are always given capital letters to distinguish them from our normal understanding of the terms.

The Child

This is the original and perhaps the central ego state, the part of us that we refer to when we speak of the "real me." It is the feeling part of our being. The Child feels all our normal emotions: hurt, anger and fear as well as their opposites, happiness, love and security. As the component that provides the drive and energy for our creative activities, it is probably the only ego state observable at birth, although I believe that the other ego states are developing at this time. The Child stands before the bar of justice as the defendant in our court of the mind because only the Child ego state experiences feelings. In fact, the Child is being accused of having feelings.

The Parent

Early in life the Parent ego state develops in response to contact with people in the outside world, chief of whom are our parents. This ego state is modeled upon people in the immediate environment, the most important of whom is usually mother, since she is so close to the Child during the early learning period. This internal Parent becomes very similar to the important persons in the child's world. It merits its name since it is almost identical in thought and behavior to the true parents. A very important ego state to the individual, it provides him with a ready reference to the likely responses of the true parent. This enables the Child to know in advance what effect his behavior is likely to produce in his parent.

Each individual commences life with an instinctive feeling self. The expression of that self, the Child ego state, is very much modified by its interaction with the Parent ego state. The function of the Parent is to gather all the information it can about the people in the immediate environment of the Child so that the Child can respond in an harmonious manner to these people. The Child must get on well with these important people since it depends upon them for its survival. The Parent ego state therefore strictly mimics these people and adopts their attitudes and beliefs.

It is vitally important for the Child to maintain his parents'

38

approval and to avoid their disapproval. The internal Parent acts as an excellent means of monitoring and modifying the Child's behavior to conform with the true parents' ideas and beliefs so that it can get along well with them. The Child is aware of his great dependence upon the true parents for his very existence, and his greatest fear is that they will abandon him to his own helplessness and isolation. This possibility holds terror for the Child.

The importance of the Parent ego state can never be underestimated. Because of its sometimes hypercritical attitudes, it may be judged a negative and destructive element in the personality. This is more apparent than real because the Parent ego state primarily intends to protect the Child, although the manner in which it fulfills this function is frequently archaic and responsible for much mental ill health. The failure of many therapists to appreciate this important point has limited their understanding of the clinical problems presented to them.

At first it is difficult to accept the idea that each of us has more than one aspect to our personality. We can rather easily accept the Child ego state since most of us are aware of some of our feelings, and we can therefore appreciate our feeling self, the Child. However, it may be difficult to recognize the other ego states in ourselves, and this is particularly true with regard to the Parent.

We can perhaps more readily recognize these ego states in others than in ourselves. Children at play, for instance, are happy, sad, angry or scared, clearly in the Child ego state. At other times, as they mimic parental attitudes and behavior, they are operating within the Parent ego state. Witness the little girl playing with her dolls. She will scold them for some imagined transgression or praise them for some notable accomplishment. Further observation will reveal that she loves her dolls and cuddles them. Her behavior reveals her developing internal Parent, which has modeled itself upon her own parents. In addition, she is adopting some of her parents' attitudes towards herself and is being critical, praising, or loving of herself. Clearly her Parent is interacting with her Child.

As we grow up, these ego states are likely to become more and more unconscious so that we are no longer consciously aware of their functioning. Their vigilance will never really cease, and we will later discuss how their interaction may lead to emotional problems.

The Adult
We now come to the third important ego state that can readily be

recognized in all of us. Probably maturing a little later than the Parent, it develops from that part of the mind concerned with collecting information about the world around us and filing it away in the memory banks for future reference. Every minute of the day we are using our five senses and collecting information, which proliferates every day. This data, accumulated without prejudice, is independent of other people's opinions and beliefs, much like the other knowledge that comes the individual's way. This is in direct contrast to the Parent ego state, which is totally concerned with learning exactly how others think and feel, then recording this information.

With ample data at its disposal, the Adult ego state is similar to a highly complex computer which can and does arrive at new conclusions whenever it is presented with a fresh problem. These conclusions are based upon the immense amount of information which has been amassed over the years. An understanding of the Adult role is particularly important for the analytical hypnotherapist, who must rely upon this ego state to resolve the problems which the Parent and Child have created.

Ideally, all three ego states should be acting together in harmony for the greatest well-being of the individual. It is the prime objective of analytical hypnotherapy that this ideal state ultimately be reached by the patient engaging in therapy.

These three ego states are present in all of us. They can best be understood as three separate points of view which step forward whenever a situation requires a definite course of action. The Child ego state within us will have a definite feeling about the situation, often expressed as a like or a dislike. This ego state will often express its feelings with such emotive words as "I like" or "I want," or the opposite, "I don't like" or "I don't want."

The Parent ego state, as we have said, is very concerned with what others expect and want, and it utilizes words that indicate this concern. When we find ourselves saying such things as "I ought" or "I should" or, alternatively, "I ought not" or "I should not," we are using phrases that express our concern for other people's expectations of us. We are using our Parent ego state. This ego state also comes into play when, like the little girl with the dolls, we counsel, advise or criticize others in a parental manner, or whenever we take responsibility for others.

When operating from our Adult viewpoint, we are either giving information in a purely factual manner or presenting conclusions that we have reached from information in our possession. We say things like "I can" or "I will" or "it is"; we may offer the opposite statements of fact or intention, e.g., "I cannot," "I will not" or "it is not."

From the foregoing I trust that you now accept the premise that you are not just one person with a single point of view. You carry within you more than one point of view about any given situation, and these viewpoints can declare war upon one another. Consider how quickly a Child's "I want" may clash violently with the Parent's "I should not." Incidentally, this is the basis of much Parent/Child conflict, of which we shall have more to say.

Now that we have been introduced to the three ego states, which all of us possess, it is possible to consider the role that each plays in the continuing drama of the court of the mind.

The Accused

The accused is always the Child, the central part of the personality that is being prosecuted for a feeling or some other attribute that has caused offense. For example, the Child may have been accused of existing, of being a girl or a boy, or even of having certain unacceptable human feelings such as fear, anger or hurt.

The Prosecutor

The prosecutor is usually a parent, more probably mother than father. Mother is the more likely to be affected by any of the accused's (the Child's) attributes since she is in close daily contact with him. Siblings, grandparents and teachers can also function as prosecutors. The accuser is always someone within the Child's immediate environment who has been distressed by who he is or something he has done because of who he is.

The manner in which the prosecutor communicates his distress may vary considerably, but whatever method is used, there is no doubt left in the Child's mind that he is considered entirely responsible for the distress caused to the prosecutor.

The Judge

The unenviable task of Judge falls to the Parent. Why? Because the Parent functions to prevent the Child from alienating himself from the true parent. This must be avoided at all costs. The Parent must therefore judge whether the accusation is indeed correct and whether the prosecutor is sufficiently distressed to consider withdrawal of his support and caring. The Parent must also determine whether a punishment should be imposed which will prevent the recurrence of the offense.

The Judge may be called upon to make a very rapid decision or to postpone judgment until one or more similar accusations have been made and it becomes clear that alienation of the parent is likely.

The Defense

Since there are two sides to every question, in the court of the mind the case for the defense is always fully considered.

The Child speaks up in his own defense, and his testimony is simple: he was only doing what seemed right to him. He was just being himself. This seems to him a totally adequate defense. If pressed, he might also plead that he did not know that being himself was a crime or that it would distress anyone.

Unfortunately, ignorance of the law is not an adequate defense in any legal system. The fact that the Child did not know that being himself could be considered a crime avails him nothing. His weak defense is laughed out of court. The onlookers in the gallery—friends, relatives, peers—become hysterical. How could any Child think that being itself could serve as a defense. That is unthinkable!

All is not lost, however. What about the Adult? What can he offer in defense? Unfortunately, the accusations are usually made before the Adult has gathered enough information about the world to be of much help. He, too, is acutely aware of the Child's dependence upon the parent and may confirm that the Child still lacks the physical and emotional strength to survive the hazards of the world without the help of the parent. He may reinforce the Child by assuring him that he is not abnormal and that others with the same attributes are not considered criminals for possessing them. But this support is usually quite minimal.

The Verdict

When the court retires to consider its verdict, it may spend a considerable time in reaching it or decide in the fraction of a second.

A proportion of these verdicts are "not guilty" verdicts. We do not need to consider these since no problem will arise. Verdicts of "guilty," however, will greatly concern us in this book.

When the judge—the Parent—has found the Child "guilty," he must pass a sentence which will ensure that the crime will not recur. Whatever decision the Parent now makes must be acted upon by the

Parent ego state. In the court of the mind, the punishment is always fashioned to fit the crime, and many years later, as we analyze the punishment which the Child is undergoing, we may hazard a guess at the crime that he was accused of committing.

Sometimes the sentence is not immediately administered but is held over the accused's head as a threat. We shall consider this in more detail when we look more closely at the freedoms available to the accused.

The Emotions

All creatures are responsive in some way to harmful stimuli. Human beings are no exception. Possessing the ability to be aware of injurious agents, we translate this awareness into hurt. Whenever we feel hurt, something is causing or threatening damage to us. Our awareness of hurt is so sensitive that it enables us to discern the danger even before it happens. That detection of danger can produce the response of fear, which is the feeling we get when the body is preparing itself to evade a destructive force.

Sometimes it is not possible for the individual to escape the danger, so the body has developed a further protective mechanism— anger. This state of body and mind occurs when danger must be faced and repulsed. All the aggressive fighting instincts are mobilized at this point. The objective of the anger is to either frighten the danger away or destroy it.

Thus three principal emotions protect us from danger and enable us to survive. (1) Hurt is the awareness of pain and the presence of danger. It has its human counterpart in sadness—the continued awareness of hurt. (2) Fear, deriving its strength from the memory of pain, prompts the individual to avoid further pain by fleeing its source as quickly as possible. (3) Anger protects the individual from danger either by scaring it away or annihilating it.

These three emotions—hurt, fear and anger—are often rapidly interchangeable. It would seem, however, that hurt always precedes the other two emotions, which are stimulated in direct proportion to the hurt that antedates them. Thus intense anger is preceded by intense hurt, or intense fear is always preceded by intense hurt. These emotions may be deeply unconscious, we must remember, and never present in conscious awareness. They are there at birth and presumably are present before birth. Some of the cases that I have dealt with give strong support to such a notion.

All of these emotions belong to the Child ego state, and we have

43

already seen how his expression of normal human emotion can be considered criminal.

The newborn baby is able to express its pain by crying. This usually results in the early arrival of help from his mother, who is able to locate the source of discomfort and deal with it. For the newborn the expression of pain is a cry for help. Sadness and the expression of hurt by an adult is equally a cry for help.

As the child grows older, at times help is not immediately forthcoming, and thus the pain or the threat of pain remains. At that moment the reaction of fear will occur, often by a more shrill and piercing outburst. If he is old enough, he will run to mother, who for him represents security. When he reaches mother, he will feel safe and secure. She will take care of whatever is frightening him, removing the source of any pain or hurt. Persistent fear in the child or the adult is due to this effort to find security.

The response of fear may not be adequate to obtain the security that the individual seeks. It may then be necessary for him to deal with the danger himself, transmuting his fear into anger. This may happen very quickly indeed, and many angry people are never aware of the fear that has preceded their anger. They are certainly not aware of the hurt that preceded the fear. If the individual is successful in dealing with the danger by the use of anger, he will once again feel secure. It now becomes evident that the emotions are the devices by which the individual endeavors to obtain the security essential for his continued survival.

The basic emotion, that of hurt, has as its opposite the feeling of pleasure and comfort. The individual experiences this feeling when he no longer senses any discomfort and everything seems to be at peace. For the young child or infant, mother is associated with these feelings.

The second emotion, that of fear, also seeks to achieve security and safety, and once again the infant or child associates these with the mother. Feelings of security are the antithesis of fear.

The third emotion, anger, has as its antithesis love. While dealing with danger by the use of anger, the individual, whether child or adult, is unable to feel love. Once he has resolved the danger, he can once again experience security and thus regain the emotion of love. Remember, problems occasioned by fear and hurt must be resolved before love can be established.

We have considered three primary emotions as necessary for the proper detection of and defense against danger. The question now arises, what happens when the danger, the source of hurt, is mother herself, who normally guarantees security and repose? The answer to

44

this question provides the key to the basic conflict central to all emotional disorders.

When mother is the source of hurt, the Child cannot express that hurt to her, for she will only increase it. He cannot run from her and utilize his emotion of fear to escape since he no longer has a refuge. He cannot use anger to intimidate or destroy her because he needs her for his survival. There is only one course of action open to him: he must block those emotions. He simply must not feel them.

The Parent ego state serves to repress feelings whose expression will involve the risk of parental abandonment. We have seen how the display of emotion can be regarded as a crime. We can now understand how the repression of emotion that meets with parental disapproval is the only possible recourse. The Parent ego state not only punishes the Child ego state for the crime of distressing his real parent but also protects him by preventing him from being exposed to further disapproval.

We shall see in the next chapter how the Parent in its role of judge imposes appropriate punishment and in its subsequent role of jailor ensures that the punishment is meted out.

Chapter Four

The Sentence

"The verdict: GUILTY AS CHARGED."

The time has arrived which the accused has been dreading. He has been found guilty of the crime for which he had been charged and now waits for the judge to hand down the sentence of the court.

During the trial the prosecutor has painted the accused and his crime in the worst possible colors and has demanded that he receive the maximum punishment prescribable by law. The judge, of course, has the right to consider any mitigating circumstances, and it is the prerogative of the defense to draw his attention to these.

The sentence is intended to teach the criminal through punishment that his crime will not be countenanced by his peers. The criminal will be isolated from society so that he can no longer become a threat to it. He is set up as an example to others so that they might learn that crime cannot be tolerated by society.

A judge must consider all the evidence before arriving at the appropriate sentence. He will also have to take into account the accused's previous criminal record.

In the court of the mind, the Parent, in the role of judge, has been appointed to protect a representative society consisting only of the accused and the prosecutor. His prime objective is to protect these participants from each other. In most cases the sentence that he imposes will be based very closely upon the demands made by the prosecution.

The punishment is usually made to fit the crime. If an expression of feeling has been found unacceptable, the Parent may well decree that the accused be sentenced to withhold any expression of that forbidden feeling.

The Parent must enforce whatever sentence is handed down by the court of the mind. His role then switches to that of jailor. Throughout the prison sentence the relationship of Parent and Child will be markedly affected by this jailor/prisoner relationship, which forms the basis of the continuing Parent/Child conflict. It is the cause of much emotional ill health.

You must not exist

As we noted earlier, the worst crime that the Child can be

accused of is that of existing. It is the Parent's duty to enforce this sentence. Ironically, an ego state which serves to protect the Child from the real parent must become the instrument of the real parent in subduing the Child. But the actions of the Parent ego state appear necessary. Without its intervention the greater disaster of abandonment by the real parent is seen as a strong possibility.

The sentence "You must not exist" is more common than anyone previously realized. Analytical hypnotherapy, with its unique ability to locate attitudes and feelings present at a very early age (e.g., at birth or even in the prenatal period), has enabled hypnotherapists to discover the presence and the effect of this sentence in many cases.

In carrying out the sentence, the Parent ego state usually is forced to make a compromise which is acceptable to the prosecution. When the sentence is imposed—usually at birth or shortly thereafter —the Parent ego state is unable to carry such a sentence to its logical conclusion. It can, however, make life unenjoyable and cause the Child to seek insignificance so that, for all practical purposes, he does not exist. Unfortunately, on many occasions the compromise appears insufficient and the full sentence, "You must not exist," is literally carried out. We shall consider this situation in more detail later on.

Martin was in his late thirties when he came to see me about his drinking. He did not know what drove him into alcoholism, but he was certain that it had something to do with tension because he often felt wound up before one of his drinking bouts.

Martin had great difficulty in relating to people. He was shy and lacked self-confidence, deliberately avoiding situations in which he might be thrown into contact with new people because he felt awkward and tongue-tied. His conversation in such instances was virtually monosyllabic. He was always relieved when such interchanges came to an end, allowing him to retire to some quiet corner and remain unobserved.

He had a clerical job in which he felt quite safe since it demanded little contact with the public. He took the position after leaving high school, knowing that such an occupation afforded little chance of promotion but accepting this as his lot without complaint. He was a good worker, so his job was secure.

Martin was totally non-assertive, never doing anything to upset anyone. He had few friends, and no one really close to him. He called himself a loner, and I have never met anyone who better fitted that description.

Martin explained that he had been put up for adoption shortly after birth, a fact he had not known until he reached his teens. The information had not bothered him unduly, for it had not come as a surprise. He hastened to assure me that this did not preclude any problems arising between him and his adopting parents. He loved them dearly, and he was certain that they loved him, but they were greatly distressed by a drinking problem which he felt powerless to terminate. Having heard that hypnosis was useful for helping people to relax, Martin felt that relaxing might help him to control his drinking.

In hypnoanalysis we early discovered that his mother did not want him even before he was born. He sensed a strong feeling of rejection from her. He later recalled his birth experience and was aware that, shortly after birth, his mother was unconscious. He felt totally rejected, certain that he was guilty of the worst crime in the book—he existed. When his Parent ego state judged him guilty, he was sentenced to not existing.

Martin's failure to assert himself in every sphere of life was totally consistent with the punishment he was sentenced to for daring to live. His alcoholism was the result of an attempt by his Child ego state to numb the immense pain of unexpressed hurt caused by his sensation of rejection. His Parent ego state accepted the symbolic death of drunkenness as a means of atonement for daring to live.

Therapy was long and arduous, but eventually his Parent ego state was persuaded to relinquish its duty as jailor and accept a more protective and supportive role. Martin was then able to live a fuller life. Best of all, he could leave his days of inebriation behind him.

The sentence "You must not exist" can be imposed at any time during life. I well remember another alcoholic who had survived a plane crash in which his best friend was killed. Unconsciously, the alcoholic accepted responsibility for his friend's death, but only after many years of productive living did his Parent ego state decide that the time had come for him to be put to death slowly via alcohol.

I also recall Lorne, who came to me at the age of nineteen. He wanted help with hypnosis to become more effective in his career as a musician, for his performances were deteriorating markedly. Since leaving school, he had become concerned with the deficiencies in his education and was striving to increase his knowledge. Lorne's greatest problem, however, was an inability to concentrate.

He admitted that he was not strongly self-assertive, but he attributed this to an inferiority complex which made him feel that he was not as good as any of his peers. This sense of inferiority kept him from establishing relationships with women. His life was a lonely one.

Lorne recalled that he had been miserable at school, which he gladly left after completing grade ten. But now he often felt depressed

49

and was positive that he was no good—and that he would never be any good. Life did not seem to be worth living.

In hypnoanalysis Lorne regressed to a frightening experience at the age of four years when he almost drowned. He relived this episode with a great deal of distress, which he had never previously expressed, even recalling the fear on his grandfather's face as he pulled Lorne from the water. Lorne had decided that anyone who could cause such distress did not deserve to live. From that moment he shut himself away from the life which his Parent had decided he did not merit. He was eventually able to reverse this decision and at last achieve the objectives that he sought.

You must never feel angry

Anger is a way in which we defend ourselves against hurt, and the energy of that anger is directly proportional to the hurt or fear which engendered it. Anger is a natural defense which is instinctively present in the Child. Each of us learns in his own way how to use anger most effectively.

In the learning process the Child may express his anger clumsily and in doing so may inadvertently threaten and frighten those upon whom he depends for sustenance and security. If their response to the Child's anger is extreme, he is liable to become convicted of the crime of being angry. Because he has shown himself unable to manage his anger, the Child is sentenced by the Parent to shun anger. This can be translated as "You must never feel angry."

The repression of a normal defense by the Parent is a common cause of many emotional illnesses and of a high proportion of psychosomatic ailments. I have already given some examples of this mechanism, but let me add one more.

Jane was a forty-year-old woman who was plagued by severe headaches. After thoroughly subjecting the problem to intense investigation, her physician concluded that no organic cause existed. When she first consulted me, Jane was experiencing a severe attack almost every week. She frequently had to retire to bed and was unable to join in family functions or social outings.

Between attacks Jane felt healthy but lethargic and subject to depression. She said that she would not mind the depression so long as she did not suffer terrible headaches.

We discussed her attitudes toward herself and life in general. She did not consider herslf a very good person, although she tried very hard to be one. She always did what she felt people expected of her.

50

If her sister called her to come and baby-sit, for instance, she complied without complaint. If her mother wanted to visit, she was welcome at any time because Jane would always stop whatever she was doing or planning in order to accommodate her. She knew that her children made too many demands upon her, but she felt that she must always do her best to be a good mother. She also worked hard to please her husband and believed that if it were not for her headaches, she would have been as good a wife as she wanted to be.

In hypnoanalysis we discovered an important experience which had determined her attitudes. At the age of five Jane had quarreled with her younger sister, who had deliberately pulled an arm off Jane's favorite doll, even though she had been told not to play with it. Jane struck her sister forcefully. Naturally, her sister screamed loudly, and before long mother came running to discover the cause of the commotion. Jane told mother the truth, but instead of winning praise for having disciplined her sister, Jane became the object of her mother's wrath. Mother struck Jane sharply and sent her to her room, ordering her never to hit her sister again.

Jane had never been able to express her anger since that incident, and until she sought help for her headaches, she was totally unaware that that event had precipitated the problem. She was then able to recall many instances when she had felt unfairly treated but had repressed her emotions. She had been condemned to the prison of anger, unable to feel or be angry. But she could entertain headaches!

Migraine is a silent screaming in the head. Once Jane found that she could allow herself to scream out loud, she no longer needed to scream silently and her headaches disappeared. If ever a hint of a migraine arises, she immediately gets in touch with the anger she is holding back and finds means of expressing it appropriately, whereupon her headache invariably disappears.

You are not lovable—you are BAD!

The pain of rejection is acute and intense. The greater the need for acceptance, the greater the hurt of rejection. Thus the repudiation of the Child by his mother creates in him the gravest hurt, and it is not assuaged by the natural conclusion that the Child is rejected by his mother simply because he is unlovable.

"You are not lovable" is the sentence delivered by the Parent to the Child who has committed the crime of asking to be loved by a mother who is unable to love him. The sentence must be served in the prison of pain and sadness, with the added restriction of "You must not feel sad" and the burden of the accusation "YOU ARE BAD!"

Susan was thirty-three years of age when she came to me for help in controlling her eating habits. Frequently depressed and exhausted, she could not locate the source of her depression, but she admitted to being constantly tense. She found it very difficult to enjoy life and felt inferior to her friends and acquaintances. She was always irritable with her family and expressed remorse for this. When Susan came for treatment, she was certain that stronger dieting will power would solve most of her problems.

In hypnoanalysis she uncovered several experiences in which she had made attempts to persuade her mother to express love for her. Each time she met with a rebuff.

At three years of age, for instance, young Susan rushed in from the garden with the lovely flowers that she had picked for her mummy. Instead of being met with loving appreciation, she was thrust away with "You naughty girl, Susan." This was her first experience with rejection.

When she was about six years old, she had completed a lovely painting especially for her mummy. When she entered the house, all excited about presenting the painting, her mother took one look at it and snapped, "Put that mess in the garbage."

She could never persuade mother to love her. When her mother died during Susan's twentieth year, the girl was still trying to gain her love. Susan could not accept this defeat because she believed that until her mother professed love, she was unlovable. This was the frightful sentence that she had to serve, and was only terminated after a great deal of therapy.

You must not succeed

At a conscious level everyone wishes to be successful. Success, the symbol of public recognition and acceptance, is one of life's most pleasant experiences.

Sometimes, however, acceptance in one area will result in rejection in another. Under such circumstances acceptance and success can be considered a crime, punished by the sentence "You must not succeed." This judgment may be imposed upon any criminal locked within the prison of guilt. When the Child is safely imprisoned, he may be allowed to become enthusiastic about any number of projects, but should he approach any degree of success, the Parent will bar him from it so that he fails.

James labored under this sentence. He had done well at school in his early years but quit at the age of sixteen without any documentary evidence of his ability. He worked at several jobs for a while, then decided to start his university career as a mature student. After an initial burst of enthusiasm, his studies rapidly fell apart, and he left the university before completing the first year.

Since then, James had worked in several different jobs, but the same pattern continued to repeat itself. He would always become very excited about a new job and would do extremely well for a few weeks. His new employer would be very pleased with the young man who worked so diligently and was so full of new ideas. But at the end of several weeks or at the very most a few months, when his boss might be considering permanent employment, James would lose his enthusiasm, acting in ways that would usually ensure his dismissal— arriving late for important assignments, forgetting appointments, starting to drink heavily. Eventually he would be sacked—or he would quit when he felt that he had given his boss a hard enough time.

During this period his original enthusiasm would be replaced by depression and irritability. Once he left a job, his spirits would gradually lift, and although he would always feel guilty about having loused up another chance, his depression would fade. Because James was such an intelligent young man with many excellent ideas and, of course, plenty of experience, he was usually able to secure a new job and start the same cycle once again.

When he had undergone psychotherapy during a previous bout of depression, the astute psychiatrist had pinpointed the age of four years as a time when something had happened to James to cause his problems. Unfortunately, the psychiatrist had not been able to move further. In hypnoanalysis we were able to locate the experience and bring it to consciousness. At four years of age James had been surprised by his father in a sexual act with an older boy. He had been punished severely by his father but had repressed the whole experience from his memory. The intense guilt, however, remained with him. He had been exiled to the prison of guilt with the sentence "You shall not succeed."

James could not achieve success until he was freed from the prison. Till then his Parent would not let him fully exercise his abilities. He was not good enough.

You must not be afraid

Fear is a normal human response to real or imagined danger. Unfortunately, many parents do not understand fear and are disturbed by it when they perceive it in their children. In addition, society frequently interprets normal fear as cowardice. For these reasons fear may be viewed as a crime, and the Parent is given the task of ensuring that it is not repeated by passing the sentence "You must not be afraid."

An emotion that is blocked by the Parent in this way is often expressed in some more acceptable way. Overeating, excessive smoking, alcoholism and some psychosomatic illnesses can result from the repression of fear.

Elizabeth was a tall, stately girl of about twenty-eight years of age. She had separated from her husband after a short and stormy marriage several years before she came to consult me. She overate and felt constantly irritable, and her symptoms had become much worse since she had heard that her husband was back in town. He had been away for many years, and she really had no wish to see him again. He had failed to provide support for their eleven-year-old son or her since their separation.

In hypnoanalysis Elizabeth regressed to a stormy incident which had occurred when she was eighteen years of age. Her husband, in a drunken state, was yelling violent abuse at her. She was crying, the baby was screaming, and the dog was barking—a terrifying commotion. She clamored for her husband to leave her alone, and he did so for a few minutes. When he returned, he was brandishing a shotgun which he assured her was loaded. She was now even more terrified but knew that she must not lose control. She pleaded with him to put the gun down, but he ignored her, accused her of infidelity and shouted that she did not deserve to live. He was determined to kill her. As she pushed him and the gun away, the dog jumped up at him. She fled to a neighbor's house, but as she ran, a shot rang out. Had he killed himself? Had he killed the dog? The baby?

With these thoughts running through her head, she felt enormous guilt that she had left in a panic. She knew that she dared not go back lest she become the next victim, so when she became sufficiently coherent to convey to her neighbor the urgency of the situation, the police were called in.

When the police arrived, they found that nothing untoward had occurred. Uncovering no evidence that a shot had been fired, they gave her the distinct impression that they did not believe her story. They assumed it had really been an ordinary domestic quarrel in which no one's life had ever been in danger.

Shortly after this incident Elizabeth left her husband despite his threats to "get her." She had not allowed herself to think of the experience since that time, and even now, knowing that he had returned to the neighborhood, she did not connect him consciously with her symptoms. She only knew subconsciously that she must not be afraid.

You must not love

Everyone will agree that loving is a perfectly normal human emotion, yet many people are unable to express it because of a sentence imposed upon them. They have been found guilty of loving and have been sentenced never to love again. Loving is often confused with sexual activity, so that this inability to love is accompanied by an inability to enjoy sex. This may be expressed as a fear of relishing or being involved in sex. Making oneself unattractive is one way of avoiding sex and denying love.

I well remember Freda who, at twenty-three years of age, would have been quite attractive had she not been grossly overweight. She had never dated. She felt compelled to eat, almost as if she was afraid to lose weight. In hypnoanalysis the reason for this became clear.

At five years of age she was awakened by the noise of her parents quarreling violently. Freda tried not to listen, but she could not help overhearing her mother scream, "Why don't you have her? You want her more than you want me!" She wondered, could mother be referring to me? She felt sure that she loved her daddy more than her mother did. As she listened, one accusation both frightened and puzzled her. "You like little girls too much. Next time they will lock you up for life!" When she heard that, she knew that she must not allow herself to think loving thoughts about her daddy ever again. She must not love, for loving is a crime. She knew then that if she became as fat as Mrs. Johnson next door, whom daddy hated, she would be safe. She would simply eat and eat. She must supplant love with eating.

It was a long time before Freda could feel free to reverse her decision and let herself lose weight. She had to learn that it was permissible to love.

You must not think

To be considered stupid would normally be deemed a handicap, but sometimes it is wiser to act stupid than to use one's normal intelligence. Being intelligent has, on occasion, proved to be so disastrous that it has been interpreted as a crime. The proper punishment for such a crime is, of course, "You must not think."

55

I can best illustrate this through the experience of Stewart, who came to see me at the age of nineteen. He was doing very badly in his studies, finding it difficult to concentrate upon academic assignments and wondering whether he should drop out of high school rather than continue to work toward graduation.

Stewart was feeling very nervous and was unable to sleep. Only infrequently could he relate to his classmates, most of whom were younger and better students than he. However, until he had reached grade six he was scholastically ahead of his contemporaries and was the youngest and brightest in the class. He had no idea why his performance in school had deteriorated so badly since then.

We discovered the clue in hypnoanalysis. Stewart located a critical experience at the age of eleven years. He had not been in bed for long when he heard a loud bang coming from downstairs. His parents had just returned home, quarreling vehemently, his father shouting abuse at his mother. He was not sure he had caught one statement accurately, but his father shortly repeated it: "I always knew he wasn't my kid—he's too smart-assed!"

Stewart loved his dad, and he wanted no one else for a father. ·Being smart must be a crime, he decided, so he must be punished. He must not think. From that time onward, although the incident was never mentioned, Stewart began to do poorly at school. He could not allow himself to perpetrate the crime of being smart and run the risk of losing dad.

Chapter Five

The Prison Locks—GUILT!

Central to the whole theme of this book is the conflict between the Parent ego state and the Child ego state, which so often leads to the imprisonment of the Child by the Parent.

Although every prison has its jailors, they would not be so effective if the prison were not securely locked. It is natural to wonder how the Parent is able to prevent the Child from escaping. The answer is guilt, which provides locks secure from tampering.

Although all of us have experienced feelings of guilt, it is very difficult, to define the exact nature of guilt. We would all agree however, that guilt feelings are intensely unpleasant because they remind us that we have done something which has met with intense disapproval.

There is no inborn sense of guilt. It is a learned response resulting from an awareness of having been responsible for another's distress. Our acquaintance with this feeling begins when we first witness the distress of someone upon whom we rely for support and protection. That person is usually mother, and we are soon aware of our responsibility for her distress by indications that her anger is directed at us. Immediately we admit to the crime.

Even though we may not know the extent of our crime, we know that it must be something terrible because of the severity of the distress associated with it. Having been found guilty of committing a crime, we suffer grievously and may even shed tears. Mother is angry or sad or afraid, and her whole attitude verifies that we are the source of the problem. Even though we did not wish to cause distress, we are not absolved from the responsibility we feel. We sense that only a terrible person could have occasioned such catastrophic results.

The feeling of guilt emerges immediately after one has been made to feel badly and has been found guilty of one of the many crimes already listed. Guilt creates severe discomfort and is compounded of various emotions, the chief of which is fear. The basic fear is that rejection by mother will amount to total abandonment by her. Although guilt is primarily a feeling of fear, it is compounded with feelings of sadness as one contemplates the possibility of being utterly alone.

This fear potentially gains its strength from an instinctive awareness probably founded on the memory of a total dependence on her during intrauterine life, that life without mother can be equated with death. I think that the infant is aware of his dependence on mother, particularly when she does not promptly meet his many demands. He is left with a frightening sensation of helplessness since he is unable to satisfy his own biological needs.

Throughout pregnancy mother has provided continued biological support, and for us all the separation from mother at birth is a traumatic reminder of our dependence upon her. Therefore any threat of a more permanent separation from mother always becomes the source of intense fear, which supplies the feeling of guilt with its immense power.

The Parent ego state acts to prevent mother from withdrawing support from the Child by initiating a behavior pattern which is acceptable to her. This is why the Parent ego state is so closely modeled upon mother or other parental figures upon whom the Child depends for sustenance. It also explains why the Parent ego state imposes restrictions upon the behavior of the Child through the mechanism of repression. I believe that the feeling of guilt provides that mechanism.

Whenever the Child wishes to express a feeling that might produce parental disapproval, the Parent flashes the memory of the original crime with its accompanying threat of punishment by abandonment of the Child by the mother. The memory of that threat fills the Child with foreboding and provides the essence of the feeling which we call guilt.

Guilt, then, resides at the center of the Parent/Child conflict. It is the pressure applied by the Parent in opposition to and in response to the pressure of the unacceptable emotion which the Child wishes to express. Guilt effectively holds the Child in his prison and serves as the locks on the doors of the outer walls of his prison.

Intense guilt is felt as anxiety. Lesser levels of guilt may be experienced as feelings of shame or embarrassment. Although always present in cases of Parent/Child conflict responsible for imprisonment of the mind, guilt may not reach awareness and sometimes can only be identifiable at an unconscious level in hypnosis.

It is the objective of hypnotherapy to pry open the locks of guilt so that the Child may be free to express himself as he is. Before this can be accomplished, however, the Parent must be convinced that it is no longer necessary for the Child to be locked up in the mental prison for his own protection. Since the Parent ego state regards the prison as a haven of security as well as a place of punishment, it must be assured that the Child will not come to far greater harm should he be released. An understanding of this function of the Parent enables us to accept its very important role as the purveyor of guilt in the interests of the individual.

Chapter Six

Release From Prison

The Appeal

The legal systems of most civilized societies contain provision for the review of a sentence imposed upon the alleged criminal after the trial. This mechanism also provides for a re-examination of the circumstances of the crime in order to determine whether the actions of the prisoner were truly criminal. The appeal procedure is designed to ensure that justice is upheld and that any evidence not accessible at the original trial can be made available to the court for its deliberation.

All successful therapy involves a review of the problem to find new and more satisfactory solutions. This approach is crucial to success in the analytical hypnotherapy of emotional problems.

Early Parent/Child conflicts often continue unresolved throughout the lifetime of the individual. The Adult remains a helpless and uninformed spectator of the painful struggle between the oppressed and miserable Child and the unyielding, duty-conscious Parent. Neither Child nor Parent is able to communicate the true nature of the conflict to the Adult in order to allow this highly resourceful ego state to discover a solution to their conflict. Internal communication is clearly inadequate. When psychotherapies work, they probably do so simply by utilizing Adult understanding of the Parent/Child conflict so that the Parent can be supplied with the information necessary to moderate its position and allow the Child increased or full freedom.

Successful therapy operates in the same way as an appeal. Grounds for the appeal may include the following: that the original trial was conducted ineptly, that the sentence given was too severe or that new evidence is now available to the court.

Before an appeal can proceed, a report of the previous trial must be made available to the defense for study, largely because the memories of the original event which precipitated the emotional conflict are no longer present at a conscious level. They are often not available to the Adult even at an unconscious level because the Adult ego state was probably too immature at the time of the original event to form an understanding.

In the recovery of unconscious memories hypnosis possesses a unique advantage over all other therapeutic approaches. I would suggest that any approach which incorporates communication with the unconscious mind is in fact using hypnosis. Hypnotic techniques are being employed successfully by many therapists who are not aware that hypnosis is involved and who have no formal knowledge of hypnosis. This statement in no way detracts from the merits of these successful techniques but seeks to recognize and identify the common pathway necessary for success.

Analytical hypnotherapy depends upon direct communication with the unconscious mind for its ability to locate information regarding the original problem. Fortunately, we have found that for most people adequate communication with the unconscious mind is relatively easy and that a deep state of hypnosis is not necessary, as was once thought. Many of my patients, in fact, are amazed at the ease with which this communication with the unconscious mind can be established, even when the conscious mind is observant and alert.

The unconscious mind is like a video tape recorder, transcribing every significant happening in faithful detail. The first step in analytical hypnotherapy is to locate the memories of the experiences from which the so-called crime and the subsequent sentence arose. The techniques of analytical hypnotherapy direct the unconscious mind to search its millions of recordings until it locates the relevant critical experiences.

The next step is to bring that experience to a level where it can be reviewed by the Adult ego state. Sometimes this experience is too painful to be brought to a conscious level and must be examined by the Adult at an unconscious level only. I have found, however, that this may be just as effective as a review of the experience at a conscious level, but it is unsatisfying in some respects for the therapist, who is left in ignorance of the basic problem and cannot develop a full knowledge and understanding of it.

If a detailed review of the original trial brings forward sufficient evidence that some injustice has occurred, a retrial can be instigated. This retrial will reconsider the crime, review the evidence for the prosecution, and any new evidence for the defense.

The Retrial
At the original trial the prosecution's case rested largely upon an admission by the Child that the events described did indeed take place and that his behavior caused his parent's distress. At that time no notice whatever was taken of the Child's pleas that he could not help it.

62

The question "Were you in fact present when your mother expressed great distress at your presence?" could only be answered affirmatively. No one showed any concern with the Child's pleas that he did not know how he got there.

At the retrial the Child has a mature Adult for an advocate who can now find many precedents to aid in the defense. Convicted of the crime of existing, the Child now has an excellent defense. In short, he was not responsible for his presence in this world, and a mature Adult has ample evidence to present in support of this viewpoint. He knows the role that his parents played in his conception and realizes that his distressed mother had a far, far greater share in the responsibility for his presence than he could ever have had. She is hundreds of times more guilty than he. This is an extremely strong defense. Furthermore, mother's distress was much more influenced by social and economic factors than by the birth of the Child.

Perhaps the Child committed the crime of anger. In that case his advocate, the Adult, can produce evidence to show that all human beings experience anger and that it is a normal human emotion which can be used for benefit as well as injury. The Adult can provide evidence that anger is not in itself a crime since it is an emotion primarily designed for protection.

In further defense of the Child, the Adult can bring the same support of any normal, healthy human feelings to an outdated charge that such feelings are crimes.

During analytical hypnotherapy much of this is frequently accomplished at a totally unconscious level; the patient is not aware of what has been done and indeed may not feel very different during the process. On the other hand, uncomfortable old feelings may be re-experienced, and he may be surprised at their intensity since he probably believed that he had managed to discard these outdated feelings many years previously. The conscious reaction may well occasion the remark, "Fancy such a stupid little thing like that still making me so upset."

This review of old experiences is often accompanied by intense feelings since it requires that an event which was partly or wholly responsible for the Parent/Child conflict be examined in detail. The techniques of analytical hypnotherapy are designed to ensure that a thorough re-examination of the experience is accomplished. In fact, a session of hypnotherapy may review several such critical experiences. This initial phase of hypnoanalysis cannot be regarded as complete until all such experiences have been thoroughly examined and the deep modern understanding of the mature unconscious Adult ego state has been applied to each of them.

The purpose of this review is to persuade the Parent ego state to reverse its original verdict of guilty since this had resulted in the incarceration of the Child and the subsequent conflict between them. The Parent usually welcomes relief from the onerous duty of Jailor. On the other hand, it may find it difficult to accept the new role of friend and supporter of an ego state which for years it has held in contempt as a common criminal.

Throughout this process the Adult concentrates all of its powers of logic upon the Parent/Child conflict. This phase of analytical hypnotherapy calls for the greatest exhibition of skill and patience from the hypnotherapist. He is aware that he cannot free the Child himself but must rely upon the Adult ego state's effort to persuade the Parent to permanently release the Child.

If the Parent cannot be fully convinced that the Child is innocent or that he has been punished sufficiently, the Child will only be allowed out on probation. This is not good enough, however, for it projects only a false freedom and will inevitably be followed by a relapse after a brief period of remission. Unfortunately of course, we are sometimes forced to settle for this probation rather than the total and unconditional pardon that we seek.

The Pardon

Normally a pardon can only be obtained when a case has been reopened and irrefutable new evidence of innocence has been presented. The defendant is then considered to have been wrongly convicted and unjustly imprisoned.

A pardon is essentially a sincere official apology that an injustice has occurred. It is an affirmation that the defendant has always been totally innocent of the crime for which he had been charged and sentenced. His good name is once again restored to him, and he is regarded as a thoroughly worthy citizen who is just as respectable as any of his fellow citizens who have not undergone his unfortunate experience.

It is this kind of unconditional pardon that analytical hypnotherapy seeks to secure for the Child from the Parent. In most cases a Child has been convicted of multiple crimes, and it is imperative that a pardon be obtained for each separate crime. When this happens, many wonderful things occur—the chief of which is the Parent's acceptance of the Child. Our patient begins to like himself.

The Parent must cease to act as a controlling, repressive force and must become an encouraging and supportive one. Sometimes this is accomplished quite rapidly, but often it takes a great deal of persuasion from the logical Adult ego state to achieve a reversal of behavior. Until now the Parent's natural loving and nurturing functions have been largely subordinated to its disciplinarian role. Teaching the Parent new approaches is an important part of hypnotherapy.

A true pardon is permanent. There will never be any need for the Child to enter prison again. The Parent/Child conflict is at an end and the patient is cured. The sense of freedom experienced by the pardoned Child can only be truly understood by someone who has undergone it. We will be hearing from pardoned prisoners who will describe their escape from prison and their subsequent experience of freedom.

Freedom

Liberty is every human being's birthright. To be free is to be oneself, to express one's personality without fear or guilt. This should be the ultimate objective of all psychotherapy.

The freed Child is in harmony with his Parent ego state and can be trusted to experience his feelings fully and without hindrance from the Parent. There is no longer any conflict between the Child ego state and the Parent ego state, and there remains little for the Adult ego state to do but to provide the Child with the information necessary for him to be able to fully utilize all the creative energy of his feelings.

Thus the once unproductive artist is slowly transformed into a creative and fully productive craftsman. The shy, retiring individual becomes open and communicative. The psychosomatic ailments are no longer necessary, and the normal health which was previously concealed by these symptoms emerges. The feeling of well-being that the free Child brings to the personality is without parallel. In some cases it borders on the miraculous.

Freedom can take place quite suddenly, as we have often noted in the phenomenon of religious conversion. When it does, such an experience occurs quickly, it appears miraculous, shocking the family and friends of the convert. They must learn to adapt to the freed person, who has suddenly appeared in their midst like a stranger. This change in him, of course, may strain their adaptive powers. Until they realize that the freed individual—despite his openness—has no malicious intent and will do them no deliberate harm, they may not be able to handle him. Sometimes marriages that have not been stable will collapse when a partner is freed. It has been my experience, however, that the other partner can usually discover resources with which to deal with and adapt to this change. Accordingly, the marriage relationship will often become quite beautiful.

Usually the transformation in the freed personality is quite gradual. The Parent, persuaded to alter his role from that of Jailor to Supporter and Protector of the Child, shifts roles slowly. In such cases the family still has to adjust, but in subtler ways and over a longer period of time.

In the phase of freedom the Adult ego assumes great importance. The Child is now at liberty in a new world of free expression and is aware of emotions which were previously repressed. He requires direction from the Adult in learning ways to exhibit these emotions which will not alienate him from the community to which he aspires to belong.

Anyone who has been released from one of the mind's emotional prisons must learn how to use that newly released emotion without any sense of guilt. Anything short of this is not true freedom. The new role of the Parent ego state is so important in the establishment of the new freedom that therapy must continue until this role is fully accepted. Occasional relapses will result from a failure to establish the Parent's new role as Supporter and Protector of the Child ego state.

Chapter Seven

REHABILITATION—
Learning How To Remain Free

Our prisons are full of men and women who are unable to adapt to life in the free world. As soon as their sentences end, they commit new crimes and are reimprisoned.

Many prisoners have been isolated from normal society so long that they cannot comprehend the established rules of order and soon run afoul of them. Others return to prison because they lack the skills with which to function adequately in a free society. They are untrained to live outside of prison.

Another group of released prisoners miss the security of prison and are fearful of the demands that living in a free world imposes upon them. These prisoners may deliberately commit offenses which they know will ensure their recommittal to the safe haven of prison.

The problem of recedivism has long occupied the attention of sociologists and criminologists. It seems to be virtually insoluble, but there is general agreement that if satisfactory rehabilitation were truly possible, the problem would be greatly reduced.

Prisoners of the mind are unique among criminals because they were really never guilty of any crime. After pardon their rehabilitation becomes an extremely important problem. Prisoners of the mind must be taught to make their way as free human beings in a strange world which may be somewhat hostile to those who have newly been freed.

Two very important phases of rehabilitation must be satisfactorily completed before the prisoner can be said to handle his freedom satisfactorily. In the first phase he must be convinced that he has the right and the ability to be free. In hypnotherapy we call this process ego strengthening, for it is a procedure for increasing the strength of the Child ego state. The second phase is that of assertiveness training. It is necessary to instruct the Child and the Parent in new ways of handling the problems of life with the assistance of the Adult. When these two phases have been satisfactorily completed, the released individual is properly prepared to handle his new-found freedom.

Ego Strengthening

Until this point, hypnotherapy has been directed to locating

67

critical experiences which have made normal human feelings appear to be crimes. The Child ego state has been subjected to a punishment consistent with his crimes and has had the expression of his forbidden feelings severely restricted by guilt.

In obtaining freedom for the Child, the Adult ego state has at last been able to convince the Parent ego state of the Child's innocence. For the Parent this is a novel conception since it had previously listened only to the true parent, and this idea is apparently in total contradiction to all it had heard. This conception therefore must be repeatedly reinforced for it to be permanently accepted by the Parent.

On the other hand, the Child, although always believing in his own essential innocence, initially finds it difficult to conceive that he is acceptable. He is not completely sure that he is really O.K.

Ego strengthening is an important and essential part of therapy, and hypnosis plays a vital role in retraining both the Child and the Parent to accept and maintain belief in the Child's basic innocence and acceptability.

The effective therapist himself must possess a deeply rooted conviction of the essential goodness and rightness of human nature. The tools of hypnosis will allow him to communicate this conviction to the unconscious mind of the patient. This point of view may have to be repeated many times until the previously impoverished Child ego state gains sufficient strength to maintain the belief at all times. The Adult ego state continues to aid the Child in this belief in himself by providing him with ample information of his equality with and essential resemblance to other human beings. He can, therefore, be persuaded that he need no longer feel inferior to his fellow human beings.

By using hypnosis to secure the attention of every part of the unconscious mind, I can be certain that each ego state is listening to me. I begin by stating emphatically that every human being is important. I then ask for agreement with this viewpoint from every part of the patient's unconscious mind.

Following this, I assert that my patient is just as good and important as any other human being living or dead. I find this easy to state in a convincing manner because I sincerely believe it. If my patient has really freed himself from all punishing restrictions, he can agree with me and accept this revolutionary point of view. The belief that one is really just as good and important as any other human being is always accompanied by positive feelings.

When a patient cannot concur that his significance matches that of any other human being, I know that his Parent ego state is having difficulty in yielding its accustomed role as jailor. Partial agreement with these principles indicates that the Parent has not been wholly convinced to play a supportive role and may resume the former restrictive function at any time. At such a point we must pursue further analytical hypnotherapy for the Child to be totally and permanently free.

In order to increase ego strengthening in those who are apparently free, I always ask my patient in hypnosis if he agrees that he has a right to respect and protect his normal human emotions, whether or not they are pleasant. This question is really directed to the Parent ego state. I am inquiring whether it accepts the new role of respecting and protecting the Child and his normal human emotions. If I gain an affirmative response to this question, I know that the ego of the Child has been immeasurably strengthened by the knowledge that its feelings have been accepted. It now has the full support and protection of the Parent ego state.

Assertiveness Training

Many courses and teachings today address themselves to the subject of assertiveness training. Unfortunately, a mental prisoner cannot avail himself of the good advice contained in these writings and teachings. That is, his Parent will not allow him to indulge in self-assertion since that is a privilege reserved for the free.

When an individual fully accepts himself, however, he has no need to be particularly assertive. His respect for himself is evident, and he commands respect from others. Only those who cannot respect themselves fail to gain respect from others. It is precisely this group of people who, though needing assertiveness training, cannot avail themselves of it because they are imprisoned.

When an individual escapes from his self-imposed prison, he emerges into a strange world where no one recognizes him. At first not even his friends or relatives see him for what he truly is, for they have only known him as a prisoner. As a free person he no longer feels guilt about himself, and this very fact makes him a stranger to his peers.

To overcome this difficulty, the newly released prisoner must learn to support and protect himself in the outside world. He will be called upon many times to justify his presence outside prison walls and will have to know how to assert his right to be free.

The liberated prisoner must learn three simple things. First of all, he has to learn how to prevent his Parent from reimprisoning him.

This requires a great deal of alertness on the part of the Adult, who must constantly remind the Parent that his old role of Jailor is finished. Secondly, he must learn to rely upon the Parent ego state to protect him whenever others attempt to have him recommitted to prison. Once again the Adult must be prepared to recognize when this is happening and to call upon the Parent to ward off any such attempt in his proper role as the protector. Thirdly, he must not be seduced into any situation in which he might be tempted to use the tool of guilt upon others in order to lock them more securely within their own prisons as a reprisal for their attacks upon him. All of this requires effective assertiveness training.

Hypnosis offers an excellent medium for productive assertiveness training because suggestions given in hypnosis are attended to very closely and, when accepted, are followed with utmost fidelity. In practice, I accomplish this stage of therapy by demanding that the individual make and keep three important promises.

First, he must promise to stop putting himself or his feelings down. This is the most essential promise that I extract, for it is the most difficult to keep. Until now, the Parent has repressed the Child and discounted his feelings. If the promise is kept, the Child will receive the essential support of the Parent.

Secondly, I ask the individual to promise never again to allow anyone to put him or his feelings down. Many patients have permitted others to get away with devaluing and ignoring their feelings or calling them into question. Their tormentors have had no right to do this, but my patients have never objected to such treatment. In fact, they probably invited others to demean them. They must now put a stop to this, never allowing anyone to make them feel badly. I sincerely believe that most people do not intentionally mean to put others down, and when they are made aware of the effect of their actions on a friend they will immediately desist. In any case, the very action of informing someone that he is causing hurt seems to make it easier to keep the first promise not to put oneself down. These first two promises supplement each other in the assertiveness training process.

The therapeutic process must extract a third and final promise: that the individual never knowingly put any one else down. Imprisoned subjects are accustomed to demeaning themselves and accordingly gain some measure of comfort from their ability to do the same to others. Those whom they attack, of course, must inhabit prisons of their own to be vulnerable. Thus both sides frequently engage in useless, damaging battles. A prerequisite for disengagement from such fighting demands an "ex-convict" no longer knowingly put others down.

For each of these important assertiveness training promises the Adult ego state may be provided with an excellent rationale which it can utilize to ensure that there is always complete ego agreement. This further enhances ego strengthening. For example, the Adult accepts the Child as good and as important as any other human being, and therefore no one has the right to put the Child down—not even the Parent or Adult. It follows quite logically that neither the Parent, the Child nor the Adult has the right to put anyone else down.

This phase of therapy is administered to every patient regardless of the problem with which he first presented. If a patient can keep these three promises, he will remain free. Conversely, if he fails to keep any one of the three promises, he is in danger of reimprisonment.

This phase of rehabilitation, an essential part of therapy, is included at every visit of every patient. Each time an ex-prisoner is attacked, creating a situation in which he would formerly have remained silent and thus implicitly agreed with the attack, he now stands up for himself. He never remains undefended. His new self-confidence renders him both self-protective and self-assertive. He now respects his own feelings, thoughts and ideas, never abandoning them. Speaking up for himself, he will not allow a criticism of his feelings to go unchallenged.

Every day that the free patient deals successfully with an infringement upon his newly defined rights, he increases his self-confidence. Each subsequent defense of his feelings and opinions brings new respect from those around him and consolidates his own self-respect.

Chapter Eight

False Freedom

Many prisoners find their freedom partially or intermittently restricted for various reasons. Among prisoners of the mind we find many individuals in analogous circumstances; they are only able to achieve freedom for short periods of time.

1. Prison breaks

A prisoner can obtain temporary freedom by slipping away from his jailors when their vigilance flags. Unfortunately, he is never truly free. Always on the run from the law, he may be caught and returned to prison to face an even more severe sentence. An outlaw can never really relax. He lives in constant fear of discovery and is never free of a feeling of guilt.

In precisely the same way the enterprising Child ego state can sometimes escape the vigilance of the Parent and flee his prison. When he does so, he presents the typical clinical picture of the escapee who possesses overwhelming self-confidence. This is vastly different from his appearance in prison under the control of his jailor, the Parent.

a) The manic depressive

Typically, the manic depressive experiences periods of deep depression during which he becomes withdrawn, inactive, sad and possibly suicidal. These alternate with periods of great activity during which the patient becomes increasingly productive and creative. Unfortunately, throughout each period the patient becomes so hyperactive mentally and physically that he eventually loses control. At such times of crisis he is no longer able to think clearly or constructively. He becomes illogical and must be restrained for his own good.

The depression phase is essentially the same as any depression during which the Child is undergoing tremendous pressure from a hypercritical, punitive and restrictive Parent who tortures the freedom loving Child by constantly reminding him of his crime while meting out punishment. But if the Parent tires from the rigors of this duty and relaxes its usual vigilance, the Child can take advantage of the

Parent's absence from his post to slip out of prison.

All of us have witnessed the weary, harassed mother in the department store trying to keep an unruly three-year-old in line with threats of punishment. When she has him firmly by the hand, he cannot escape, and after a while he admits defeat and appears to become cooperative. In reality, he is simply awaiting his opportunity to escape. Eventually mother's attention is distracted by some article in the store and she releases her hold on her offspring. This is the moment he has been waiting for, and he is quick to seize the opportunity. He scampers off, delighting in his freedom, wandering from department to department, his imagination running riot as he experiments with the goodies on display.

Now one of two things may happen. If his departure is soon noted by his mother, she will give chase. In turn, he will begin to run even faster from her, although certain that she will eventually catch him, as she has done so many times before. As his speed gathers, he becomes less coordinated, and soon he falls and is apprehended. In the process he has probably made havoc among the merchandise.

But if mother does not notice his departure and quickly take up the chase, he will become lost and frightened. He will cry out for his mother, desperately seeking her protection again no matter how restrictive it proves to be.

In either case he is eventually recaptured, and his mother expresses her annoyance and anxiety at the embarrassment and fear that his excursion has caused her. She may even spank him. In any case, he will become acutely aware of her wrath and will demonstrate this by crying and sobbing. For the duration of the shopping trip he will be contrite and almost docile. He is a bad boy and he knows it.

The manic-depressive experiences a similar drama internally. The Child ego state temporarily escapes from the Parent ego state and becomes uncontrolled as the manic phase is reached. He fears both his lack of control and the probability of reimprisonment. When the Parent does again imprison him, remorse and guilt combine to render him extremely depressed.

Typically the manic depressive patient is very high in spirits in the manic phase, very low in the depressive phase. It is my clinical experience that many people undergo mood swings which, though far less dramatic than those of the manic depressive, are caused by the same mechanism. These may vary in intensity and in duration from hours to years.

This pendulum mechanism is at the root of all recurrent depression. It can only be inactivated by the intervention of the Adult ego in the continuing Parent/Child conflict. Analytical hypnotherapy is one effective way in which this can be accomplished.

Ernest is a thirty-three-year-old accountant who originally consulted with me concerning insomnia. He had not slept well for years. Sometimes he went to sleep feeling quite tired but found himself wide awake only an hour after going to bed. At other times he lay awake for hours, listening to the clock striking the early hours of the morning.

Ernest lived alone. His marriage broke down because of the demands he put upon it. When I saw him, he told me that he had experienced periods of severe depression which seemed to be heralded by a poor sleeping pattern. Only medications helped him to sleep and enabled him to combat the feelings of hopelessness and sadness which dominated these periods of insomnia.

Over the years he had been hospitalized on several occasions for periods of depression up to several weeks. Undergoing electroshock therapy on two occasions, he believed that this had hastened his recovery.

Between these periods of depression his sleeping pattern altered, he slept deeply and fairly well, although he tended to awaken early. At such times he was much more energetic and productive, by far the most effective partner in his firm. During the good periods he produced much more work than his long-suffering secretary could handle. At such times he was punctual for his appointments, drank little and devoted a fixed time each day to a fitness program.

A few days prior to each period of depression he became tense and confused. His head filled with thoughts that demanded expression, but he felt frustrated in his attempts to find sufficient creative or productive outlet. He suspected that other people were stupid because they were so slow and could not fully comprehend him. These thoughts and experiences contrasted sharply with the periods of depression which always followed.

His wife found him difficult to handle in either phase. In a state of depression he became overly dependent upon her; when he felt "well," he appeared to be under such tremendous pressure that she and the children suffered from it. He made countless family schedules for each hour of the day, but the plans were too numerous, allowing none of his family any time for themselves. When the designs began to develop, they became too complex for him to handle, and thus he would experience feelings of self-doubt. He would begin to lie awake, wondering whether he could ever be the success he was so desperately trying to be and questioning why he was so hard on everyone. In the end his wife could endure no more. She left him, taking the children with her.

His mood was already sliding downhill once again when he came to see me. If it were to continue in its usual pattern, he would soon become profoundly depressed and unable to complete even the basic responsibilities of his occupation. He would reach a stage where once again his loyal secretary would be hard put to find new excuses for her boss's incapacities.

This story took a little while to emerge in its entirety, but it was clear at our first meeting that Ernest was suffering from the destructive cycle of the manic depressive.

Having proved to be a good subject for hypnoanalysis, he regressed to a critical experience which had occurred when he was three years of age. He and his big brother Billy had arrived home late because they had played in the city park instead of coming straight home from a friend's house. Their father was in a rage when they finally arrived. He had been drinking heavily and was not in control of himself. He beat Billy unmercifully with a strap, and Ernest could only cower in abject fear awaiting his turn. But he never received his beating because father was distracted. Instead of experiencing relief, however, Ernest felt guilty and responsible for his brother's hurt.

He recalled several other events in which he was "bad"—usually lying or stealing things. In hypnosis he was able to use his Adult understanding to forgive himself for these "crimes." He realized that such episodes were part of an internal rebellion of his Child against his tyrannical Parent. His anti-social acts were not due to any malice in his character but rather represented attempts to protest the injustice of his situation.

It took quite a while for his Parent to be persuaded to accept his Child as normal and no worse than any other Child. But only when he gained the real freedom of self-acceptance did his cycles of manic depression cease.

At the conclusion of therapy Ernest was able to sleep without medication and to give up antidepressants or tranquilizers. He felt very good about himself. His work output improved and leveled off at a high but reasonable level so that neither he nor his employees were under any undue pressure. At our last meeting he related with pleasure that he and his wife were seriously considering coming together again. He was no longer depressed. His Parent ego state had at last accepted his Child and was no longer compelled to tell him how bad he was.

b) Multiple personalities

Prisoners have been known to find their way out of poorly guarded prisons and to reenter by the same route, leaving no evidence of their temporary absence. Such prisoners have excellent alibis for any offense committed on the outside, for they will be presumed incarcerated all the while.

Authorities consistently assume that their prison is escape proof. They would not even consider the possibility that a prisoner could elude their vigilance. They remain blissfully unaware that one of their charges has a method of escape and return which he regularly employs.

This would make a nice plot for a novel. In analogy, however, this is precisely what happens with some cases of multiple personality. The Child ego state has found a means of escaping the oppressive vigilance of the Parent ego state. It gets free of control in such a way that the Parent is totally ignorant of how it escapes and may be unaware that a breakout has in fact occurred.

The observer perceives that the subject has experienced a sudden change of mood or personality. But the subject suffers from periods of amnesia and only later learns that he has behaved in an uncharacteristic way. He usually describes these periods as blackouts.

Although it is not easy to understand how this rift in the personality occurs so that separate and independent personalities arise, it is always the result of great internal conflict due to the extreme oppressiveness on the part of the Parent ego state which leads the Child to formulate this unusual means of temporary escape.

When I was first consulted by Ellen many years ago, she was suffering from headaches which she had endured throughout her life. She was able to control the pain to some extent through self-hypnosis, but she came to me for analytical hypnotherapy in the hope that she could eliminate them entirely. She referred to "blackouts," during which she had little recollection of what had transpired. Afterwards she would be told that she had totally ignored the family. Engaging in a variety of artistic activities, she would become antagonistic toward her husband and quite neglectful of her normal household duties. Her "blackout," lasting for two or three days, would be followed by an intense headache. The family, she explained, eventually adjusted to her "funny moods" because she always seemed to come out of them and reassume her usual meticulous, sweet, kind and proper self.

During analytical hypnotherapy I became acquainted with a secondary personality whom I called Mary (her proper first name).

Mary informed me that she had been imprisoned by Ellen many years previously and that although she had learned to escape, she could only do so for short periods.

At these times she did what she truly wanted to do. She confessed that she did not like Ellen's husband and saw no reason why she should do anything for him. She did not even feel married to him. She admitted that she was entirely responsible for Ellen's headaches, which were imposed in retaliation for being locked up. Ellen, the Parent personality, was a perfectionist; Mary was the happy-go-lucky Child.

With the help of the Adult ego state, who was initially unaware of what was going on, we were able to arrange a kind of armistice between these two warring ego states, which eventually became friends. Therapy took quite a long time in this case, but the headaches disappeared when Mary was freed on a permanent basis. Therapy terminated when Mary Ellen became whole and peacefully united.

2. Out On Bail

When the accused is put on bail, he gives an assurance to the court that he will appear at his trial. Bail is secured when he places a monetary deposit with the court, which will be forfeited if the accused fails to return for trial. Until the trial date he will enjoy a temporary freedom. But this is a false freedom, for the accused is required to report regularly to the court and cannot travel at will.

Although he has the right to be considered innocent until proven guilty, he inevitably feels almost as uncomfortable as if he had already been convicted. On the defensive much of the time, he is constantly thinking of the forthcoming trial and the possibility of an unfavorable outcome. Furthermore, he is not certain when the trial will take place. Under these circumstances it is difficult for him to lead a normal life. He is only able to -enjoy his freedom for short periods, knowing that at any time he will be tried, perhaps found guilty and imprisoned.

All of these events may transpire in the mental life of those accused of emotional crimes. An incident occurring early in life may have all the hallmarks of an emotional crime and yet not be brought to trial until years later. It would appear as if the Child ego state had managed to buy time from the Parent ego state by promising to be good and by pleading for leniency. Charges have not been pressed at this time, probably because the victim of the alleged crime was in a forgiving frame of mind at the time of its commission.

Later in life, when the charges are laid, the Child is brought to trial and sentenced to imprisonment. At this late date the original charge is proved and the appropriate punishment administered by the Parent.

Mavis was thirty-four years of age when I first saw her for treatment of a persistent depression. She reported that she had felt depressed and hopeless ever since the birth of her son three years previously. This state had occasionally been so severe that it necessited hospitalization.

In hypnoanalysis we discovered that Mavis was four years of age when her brother was born. She was genuinely delighted by this event, for a new baby was welcome in the house and she loved the child intensely. At least she did until she began to recognize the unusual interest that her parents and her favorite grandmother were taking in the new baby. It seemed to her that they were particularly pleased that he was a boy. He drew all of the attention of the other family members, apparently because he was a boy. She felt neglected, frightened and sad. Fully aware that her brother was the cause of her hurt, one day she screamed at him, "I hate you! I hate you!" Her mother heard her discharge of anger and came to pacify her. Mavis detected the hurt in her mother's eyes and regretted her outburst. Rather than punishing her, mother picked her up and cuddled her. Right there and then Mavis promised that she would be good. In fulfillment of that promise, she never again expressed the hurt that she still felt.

When Mavis became pregnant for the first time, she desperately hoped that her baby would be a girl who would emotionally compensate her for the sister she never had and who would not be the rival that her brother had become. Her baby was a boy, however, and Mavis was terribly disappointed. She had so wanted a girl. She suddenly felt intensely guilty and began to punish herself for the crime committed thirty years earlier. She had been on bail all of these years, but now she had been tried and found guilty of hurting her mother by hating her brother—or was it her son?

Therapy helped Mavis give herself an unconditional pardon for her natural animosity toward her brother. She was at last really free. She no longer needed to punish herself by means of depression.

3. On Probation

Extenuating circumstances may often lead a court to be lenient

79

with a convicted criminal. Under such conditions he may be placed on probation, which means that although he has broken the law, he will not be imprisoned so long as he continues to behave himself. During a certain period, however, he must remain under the supervision of an officer of the court, a probation officer.

In the court of the mind a similar mechanism may be set in motion. However, the supervision period is not usually limited and thus continues throughout life. The usual clinical picture is that of an individual who in infancy experienced a traumatic emotional event which has left a very strong impression. He has dealt with this experience by a modification of his behavior which has enabled him to feel safe. This is an illusion; he is not truly safe. He is merely on probation.

I was consulted by a middle-aged physician whom I will refer to as David. He was feeling extremely depressed and did not know why. He related that he had applied for an appointment at a university since he had been assured that, because of his particular expertise, his application was likely to be successful. Unfortunately, this was not to be the case. The university to which he had applied sent him a letter of regret, explaining that they were not able to utilize his particular talents.

David was disappointed and surprised at the refusal. However, he was even more startled by his emotional reaction. In the throes of a profound depression, he felt that his life had no real meaning; he was no good. Intellectually, he knew that he was a man of great worth, but he could not feel this at all. Embarrassed by finding himself constantly in tears, he came to me with the hope that I could help him discover the cause of his melancholy.

In hypnoanalysis we soon discovered an important early experience. At his birth his mother had rejected him. She had not even wanted to look at him. This finding surprised him very much because consciously he had felt that his mother had always been very proud of his many achievements. He was ashamed of the fact that he had not been more concerned about her during her lifetime and was so little upset by her death some five years previously. Hypnoanalysis led him to a new understanding of his mother. She had not been married to his father at the time of his birth and had probably felt intensely ashamed of her unmarried status. As an infant, however, he had only been aware of her rejection, not the complex reasons behind it. He now understood that he had responded to this rejection by deciding to excel so that one day she would fully accept him. Unconsciously, however, he had never felt that he deserved her acceptance.

We uncovered a further experience which contributed to David's sense of unworthiness. At the age of four he engaged in the game of "mothers and fathers" with a little girlfriend. This is a time honored game in which children discover just how different boys and girls are. They were discovered at a crucial point of the game by the little girl's mother. The shocked tone of her voice was reechoed by his own mother's a little later, and he concluded that he could never be truly regarded as acceptable. But he knew that he must continue to try.

In therapy David was able to understand why he had always been impeled to prove himself, and he also discovered why he never seemed to derive any real satisfaction from his many triumphs. His failure to obtain the post that he had urgently desired suddenly precipitated him back into the maelstrom of maternal rejection—and all of the pain and dejection associated with it. So long as he had been successful, he had been able to remain outside the prison of pain and sadness, but his failure signalled the revocation of his probation. He was imprisoned, but with the help of analytical hypnotherapy he was able to escape.

David is now truly free. He feels that he is no longer under a compeling pressure to succeed and is pleased that he did not obtain the job that he had applied for and had wanted so much. He has moved into a related specialty in which he is happier than he has ever been.

4. Minimum Security

Not everyone in prison is closely guarded at all times. Some prisoners have day passes which allow them to work in the free world. Each evening, of course, these prisoners must return to a lightly guarded prison, but otherwise they can consider themselves free. Some of their fellow workers, in fact, may not know that their mates are prisoners, although they may be aware that these fellows avoid engagements which would keep them away from home late in the evenings.

Emotional problems operate similarly. For the victims these problems do not intrude much into their lives. At certain times, however, the victims are aware of difficulties which do not appear to have any direct connection with their experiences of the moment. They have had to return to prison.

Sara was a well-educated, self-confident divorcee in her early forties, enjoying a successful career in journalism. For some reason she occasionally went on what she called food binges. When I saw her, she looked trim and attractive, but she confided that she could put on several pounds during these binges. They frightened her because at such times she felt quite out of control, even though she usually prided herself upon her discipline and self-restraint. During these binges she would eat everything in sight until she was literally so full that she felt ill.

Sarah did not admit to having any emotional problems and could not understand why she should do this. She had been divorced for more than five years and expressed no intention of remarrying, although she had many opportunities. Her teenage children were happy and doing well at school. She was fulfilled in her work and her job was quite secure.

Sara knew these episodes of compulsive eating were imminent when she experienced feelings of panic and depression. Only when she had given way to the compulsion to overeat did her normal relaxed, cheerful mood return.

In hypnoanalysis we discovered that her apparent emotional freedom was an illusion. Her mother had been extremely disappointed in giving birth to a girl, for both parents had really wanted a boy. During Sara's childhood her father had expressed disinterest in her feminine activities but was supportive and generous with praise whenever she competed successfully in more masculine pastimes.

In therapy Sara recognized that her feelings of panic and depression developed whenever she allowed herself to become involved with a man in a sexual way. She was confined to a minimum security prison for the crime of being a woman. She could allow herself the appearance of total freedom so long as she did not become excessively feminine. Now she recognized that this restriction upon her femininity had been a major factor in the break-up of her marriage. She had never allowed herself to be sexually responsive to her husband, and this had resulted in their eventual estrangement.

Through hypnoanalysis she eventually secured total freedom from the prison of rejection and sadness and was able to enter into more meaningful relationships without the need to overeat.

5. Death Sentence

In real life, when the death penalty has been delivered for a crime, the execution is usually carried out quite soon after sentencing, although occasionally many years and numerous legal wrangles may precede its implementation. The prisoner remains in his prison cell while the legal process grinds on towards its inevitable conclusion.

During the period of waiting the prisoner may receive privileges normally identified with freedom. He can therefore foster the illusion of freedom even though he is under a sentence of death.

At times we find a patient who is laboring similarly under the sentence of death. Such people behave as if they have a death wish; their behavior is suicidal. They may take enormous risks with their lives, engage in physically dangerous occupations, drink heavily, or take high doses of drugs. They may seem incapable of making a normal recovery from a trivial illness. There are many similar ways in which the death sentence may make itself known prior to being carried out.

One would have thought that Jane commanded all the material acquisitions she needed to be perfectly happy. The envy of her friends, she had her own house and a husband who would lay down his life for her. The two young children were healthy and positively beautiful, and she herself was very attractive. At thirty she seemed to lead a life of contentment—yet she was not happy. Jane was often extremely depressed, but she concealed this so well that few of her friends could have guessed that anything was amiss. Always smiling and cheerful, Jane was laboring under a sentence of death.

Jane came to see me because she had great difficulty sleeping. She would awaken early in the morning and could not get back to sleep again, no matter what maneuver she employed. Constantly exhausted both physically and emotionally, she was impatient in her dealings with her children and her husband.

Only after a prolonged discussion of her sleeping problem did she reveal the real reason for her visit. She frequently experienced the strong feeling that she no longer wanted to live. Since her presence on earth meant little to anyone, she would not be missed if she were to die. She explained that her mother-in-law enjoyed a good relationship with the children and would be happy to care for them. Her husband would soon be besieged by a myriad of women eager to fill her vacated shoes. Her children, she lamented, would soon forget her.

I inquired whether she would want to stay alive for her own sake. She replied that she found life dull and unenjoyable; death would be a welcome release.

I soon discovered that this strong feeling of wanting to step off the edge of the world was an old one. At one time she had been strongly tempted to throw herself off a high building. At another time she took a large quantity of her mother's tranquilizers but managed to sleep the effects off without medical treatment.

Jane admitted that she did enjoy life at times, but a part of her

83

always regarded things cynically and in a detached manner. This part seemed to conclude that the whole business of living was just a chore—a gigantic waste of time. As Jane asserted repeatedly, "You are going to die some day, so why waste time hanging around?"

Although it was clear that Jane had a strong death wish, it later also became apparent that another part of her was intensely afraid that she might fulfill this wish, and for this reason she was seeking my help. Fortunately, before long we were able to discover why the sentence of death had been placed upon her.

At the age of two her older brother, the only male child, had been killed in a car accident. Many times she had heard her mother sob, "Dear God, why did it have to be the boy?" The message was very clear to the two-year-old—God had made a mistake! It should have been Jane, not Peter, who died. This message had been reinforced by her mother's complete indifference to her and her sister during a prolonged period of grief.

When Jane understood her past, she was able to get the sentence of death repealed and allow herself to enjoy life as she had a right to do. She slept comfortably and was no longer depressed.

Chapter Nine

Continued Imprisonment—
Failures of Therapy

Although analytical hypnotherapy enjoys a high success rate, there are all too many failures. Many of our triumphs, of course, had previously failed to respond to any other therapeutic approach, but so had many of our failures. In this chapter I would like to consider some reasons for these failures because I believe that much can be learned from them.

Inadequate Defense

At a trial or an appeal the defense attorney must be fully briefed on all the facts of the case if his presentation is to be effective. Sometimes the prisoner has not revealed everything that he knew about the events of which he stands accused. If cross-examination reveals that the defendant knew more than he admitted, his defense collapses. Further reopening of the case always proves to be quite difficult, requiring tremendous energy on the part of the advocate, who must be convinced of his client's innocence.

In the practice of analytical hypnotherapy the same situation can occur. The Child must locate the critical experience which brought about the original crime and divulge every aspect of the event to the Adult. If, for example, the Child has revealed that he felt hurt during an experience but concealed the fact that he was also very angry at his treatment, his advocate, the Adult ego state, may be able to persuade the Parent ego state to accept the Child's feelings of hurt as normal, but the feeling of anger will still be rejected by the Parent ego state since this has not been dealt with by the Adult. As a consequence, imprisonment continues and therapy has failed.

Until the Adult knows about the feeling of anger and can argue on behalf of the Child that this is a normal feeling, not a crime, the Parent will continue with its ordained duty of restriction and repression of the Child. Failure to secure freedom can also occur when an important critical experience is not revealed in hypnosis so that the Adult has prepared no defense whatever to the charges that are being made.

Susan initially came to me because she suffered from severe migraine headaches. They usually began early in the morning and would sometimes awaken her from sleep. We soon discovered a long forgotten experience in which she had been sexually molested by a young uncle of whom she had been quite fond. We decided that the repressed anger was responsible for her headaches because she immediately improved when she was able to express these feelings. She was delighted at this immediate improvement, but it was incomplete and, to some extent, short-lived. After a month of freedom, the headaches returned almost as severely as before.

On further examination we discovered that she had kept back a vital piece of information about the experience. She now recalled enjoying considerable pleasure during the sexual experience and was feeling guilty about her response. When she was able to accept that pleasure as a normal and inevitable response to sexual stimulation and that she did not need to be ashamed of it, she experienced further relief from her headaches. When she left therapy, I made it clear to her, as I do to all my patients, that I would be happy to see her again at any time should the need arise.

About a year later Susan came to visit me again. Her headaches had returned. She was once again bottling up her anger and her warm feelings, behaving as though she had no right to her feelings. She recognized that her headaches were a consequence of the repression of these normal responses.

At this time in my career I was beginning to realize the importance of the birth and prenatal experiences. Since I had not previously explored these with Susan, I now did so, and we discovered that her birth experience was critical. She had been the fourth girl in the family, but her parents had been desperately hoping for a boy. As she reexperienced her birth, Susan heard the doctor say, "It's another girl!" Whereupon her mother exclaimed in a disappointed voice, "Oh, no, not another girl!" To make matters worse, her father repeated these words in much the same tone. There and then she realized that she had done something quite unforgivable. From the moment of her birth Susan was on probation.

Only when Susan had passed through the second critical experience was she finally convicted of the crime of being a girl. If she had not been a girl, the molestation would not have occurred. The anger and hurt of this experience was repressed, as were any warm or loving feelings that she had experienced at the time. Her punishment was migraine.

86

Susan was now able to mobilze all of her Adult understanding in the defense of her Child. She recognized that no matter how disappointed her parents had been at her birth, she had not committed any crime by being born a girl and that this, in any case, had nothing whatever to do with her uncle's maltreatment of her. She realized that she had rejected herself and her femininity and that most of her headaches occurred whenever she was caught up in this self-rejection.

Fear of Freedom

We know that many criminals become anxious about their impending release toward the end of their sentence, primarily because they are faced with the very real problem of maintaining their social and economic independence. They understand that both of these tasks will be difficult, sometimes even insuperable. An ex-prisoner must be capable of a tremendous amount of adjustment and adaptation. If he is not, he may return to a life of crime simply to be among friends in a familiar environment. Life without them is too frighteningly isolated and lonely.

Most prisoners have experienced freedom prior to the crime that led to their imprisonment. It is very rare for a prisoner to have been born in prison, but this is precisely what has happened to many of my patients. They have never known what it is like to be free. Liberty for them carries all the fears of the unknown and is thus more frightening than anything which prison has to offer.

A significant number of patients do not want to be free. Initially they are very cooperative and appear to desire a cure. Having tried many therapies without achieving any degree of success, they blame the therapies for their failures and come to hypnotherapy as a last resort. It soon becomes apparent that they fear success when they resist any attempt to uncover the critical experience. Or if such uncovering has been successful, they will withstand any attempt to deal with it, even to the extent of discontinuing therapy on any available pretext. Such excuses as "It wasn't doing any good" or "It wasn't what I had expected." are common. I have come to respect a patient's wishes to remain in prison. He has the right to make this choice, and I no longer feel that the techniques of hypnotherapy can be held responsible for these failures. Of course, I hope that such people will eventually change their minds and decide to try life on the outside.

I have always made it clear to these patients when I have been able to reestablish communication with them that I should be pleased to resume work with them at any time, but few have accepted this offer. The prospect of freedom has been too frightening.

Inadequate Rehabilitation

In some cases our prisoners have escaped from their confines very successfully and are symptom free, but they are so ill-equipped to deal with problems imposed by freedom that they relapse. They have returned to the only security they have known, even though this means relinquishing the freedom so recently acquired. The "cure" has been short-lived; the therapy is regarded as a failure.

I can use Joan as an example. At forty-five she was an alcoholic. She had endured a very checkered life, to say the least. Her parents had separated when she was three years of age, and she and her brothers had been split up—sent to foster homes and, at one time, an institution. When I met Joan, her second marriage was on the rocks largely because of her drinking, which had created many problems for her, including a serious driving accident which had resulted in a prison sentence of several months' duration. At present she was not taking proper care of herself or of her home.

It was obvious at our first meeting that Joan was a very disconsolant, cheerless person. She was apologetic about everything that she said or did, almost as if she was apologizing for sharing the air with other people.

When I asked Joan if she liked herself, she answered with an emphatic "No." I would have been very surprised had she responded otherwise. Fortunately, she was able to enter hypnosis quite easily and quickly located her first critical moment in the birth experience.

Shortly after she was born, she heard her mother say, "I don't want his bloody kid!" She knew immediately that she had no business being born. This was confirmed later during another critical experience when she recalled hearing her mother and father in a drunken brawl fighting over her. Her father bellowed, "She's not my bloody kid!" and her mother replied, "I wish she wasn't. I wish I'd never had her at all." Shortly after this episode she began to feel very desolate and afraid, as she was being shipped off to a strange house and strange people following the final breakdown of her parents' marriage. She was now certain of her crime. She should never have been born.

Incapable of expressing the hurt to anyone, she even repressed it from herself. In hypnosis, however, she was able to get in touch with this feeling for the very first time in her life. With encouragement she was able to deal with it and relinquish it as an outdated and unnecessary feeling.

For a time all went well. She stopped drinking the alcohol she actually disliked, took care of herself and her home, and began to like herself. She felt so good that she decided to discontinue therapy. For a time she succeeded beyond her wildest dreams, but suddenly things went wrong and she turned once again to alcohol for support. She was back in prison.

When she returned to therapy, we asked ourselves, What went wrong? We soon discovered that she had not been ready for the many accusations she had to endure. The worst came from herself when she had discovered that her own daughter was heavily into drug taking— the direct result of emotional and physical damage inflicted by mother (Joan) when she was drunk. Fortunately, it did not take Joan long to recover the strong feelings of self-worth that she needed to shoulder the full responsibilities for all of her actions. Such feelings of worthiness must be well-established before rehabilitation can be regarded as complete for anyone who has been imprisoned in the jail of the mind.

I am pleased to report that Joan has experienced no further problems with alcohol and has been able to deal with many of her problems without losing any of the self-respect and self-acceptance which is vital to freedom.

Those of us who are working intensively with analytical hypnotherapy are becoming increasingly aware that it is never sufficient merely to uncover the critical experiences, deal with them and expect a permanent cure. A lasting cure can only be ensured if there has been adequate rehabilitation.

Apparent Therapeutic Failure

Not all therapeutic failures are real. In fact, some of them are not failures at all. In certain cases the symptoms for which the patient attended therapy have apparently not been eliminated, but on close scrutiny the patient does indeed feel entirely free and has resolved the problem underlying the presenting symptom. It would seem that the patient has merely altered his goals.

I have often seen this happen in cases of obesity. As hypnoanalysis proceeded, it became very clear that the question of mental freedom, not weight loss, was central. When this freedom had been achieved, the obesity became a minimal concern. Compulsive eating and the compulsive need to diet ceased. I have noted that these people have frequently lost weight gradually over the next few years.

The only way to judge the true effectiveness of therapy is to ask the patient, Are you now satisfied with yourself? If the answer to this question is an unqualified "Yes," the treatment has been a success.

Chapter Ten

The Key—
Analytical Hypnotherapy

This book is not about hypnosis. It concerns the use of hypnosis in a particular sphere of human experience—emotional distress and disorder. Hypnosis has probably been praised and decried more than any other medical treatment since it was first given notoriety by Dr. Anton Mesmer under the name of animal magnetism.

Many students of hypnosis have claimed that the process will produce marvelous cures, whereas others have countered that hypnosis simply does not exist! So long as we continue to seek for a specific state of mind which we can confidently label hypnosis, this confusion will continue and the controversy about what hypnosis can achieve will rage unabated. Hypnosis cannot and should not be regarded as a clearly definable state similar, for example, to anesthesia.

We know that when a specific dose of an anesthetic such as ether or chloroform is administered, certain predictable results occur. The patient becomes drowsy and eventually loses consciousness, no longer capable of responding to stimulation. If he is administered an overdose, he will die.

Ever since determined efforts to define hypnosis have been made, a general understanding of it has been hampered by attempts to draw parallels between hypnosis and anesthesia. This is unfortunate since there is no similarity whatever between the two. We still speak of "going under" hypnosis, even though there is never any loss of consciousness. No one goes to sleep in hypnosis, no matter how similar the conditions may superficially appear.

Many of our difficulties in understanding hypnosis have arisen from the use of it as entertainment on the stage, in novels and on television. When we witness a stage demonstration of hypnosis, we observe many phenomena which suggest that the hypnotist is exerting great powers over his subject. He appears to be able to command his subject to do anything he wishes. Many novels employ this theme of the domination of one person over another through hypnosis. We even use the word "hypnotized" to indicate a state of powerlessness.

In reality, these entertainments teach us little about the true

91

nature of hypnosis. A person in hypnosis taps the immense and largely unexplored powers of his own unconscious mind, not those of the mind of the person who administered a hypnotic suggestion. Ironically, few people have realized that this power resides within themselves, not within the hypnotist. In truth, all hypnosis is self-hypnosis.

Strange myths have been exploited and enlarged by the story teller and the stage hypnotist, but the truth is far stranger than the fiction. I hope in these pages to give you some understanding of the real wonder of hypnosis.

Human beings have achieved their dominant status in the animal world by developing the brain to encompass a far superior intelligence. Much of the brain is anatomically and physiologically similar to that of lower animals, but the cortex of the brain is so highly developed that it possesses rational qualities unmatched by any manmade computer and unsurpassed by anything known in the rest of the animal kingdom. This thinking, critical brain has developed from a far less critical but nevertheless highly complex primitive nervous system whose potential has never fully been realized.

In hypnosis the activity of this highly critical part of the brain is somewhat suspended. Hypnosis occurs naturally during great stress or whenever the deeply imaginative resources of the unconscious mind are called upon. This also happens when we are in concentrated thought. Whenever we turn to these highly imaginative parts of the mind and temporarily suspend the critical parts, we are employing the process of hypnosis.

For some reason, at present not understood, five to ten percent of the population can switch off their critical mind completely. These deeply hypnotizable people, able to accept suggestions quite uncritically, are those who have been the subject of exploitation for entertainment purposes by the stage hypnotist. They have given hypnosis a reputation it really does not deserve. Such people can readily imagine things that are suggested to them so that when the stage hypnotist tells them they are going to sleep, they simulate the act so well that they believe themselves to be asleep.

Ninety percent of the population does not possess this remarkable facility to entirely dismiss the critical faculty. Only a small minority of deeply hypnotizable subjects can switch off the conscious mind so completely that they do not recall what transpired during that period.

Fortunately for the hypnotherapist and his patients, the majority of people are able to reduce their conscious critical mental activity sufficiently to allow the unconscious imagination to function freely.

This enables suggestions to be accepted and acted upon. When they are readily accepted, we refer to the subject as being suggestible.

We must not confuse suggestibility with gullibility. The gullible person exercises a poor and inadequate critical faculty at all times, whereas the suggestible person may have an excellent critical faculty but is able to dismiss it to some degree when he so chooses.

Hypnosis is not a state but a process. It allows us to communicate ideas or suggestions to the inner and unconscious imaginative part of the mind.

By studying the ability of the very highly imaginative people who can completely dismiss the critical mind, we have been able to learn much about the potential of the unconscious imagination. It can do many wonderful things in controlling the body. For instance, it can accept the idea of anesthesia and produce its effect in a designated area of the body as powerfully as any chemical. When the unconscious mind has accepted the idea of pain relief, it can readily accomplish this. The process of communicating the idea is hypnosis.

The communication of any acceptable idea, its unconscious acceptance and the subsequent action is the process of hypnosis. By this means the tremendous resources of the unconscious mind can be tapped. At this point I would like to express my belief that the great future advances in medicine will focus strongly upon the significance of hypnosis. The unconscious mind contains vast and seemingly unlimited resources for healing which are yet to be exploited.

In this book we are concerned with the ability of the unconscious mind to uncover memories of experiences which have been recorded by the brain but retained well below the level of ordinary conscious memory. Every experience that we undergo is faithfully recorded somewhere in the unconscious mind.

Any technique which permits or facilitates communication with the unconscious mind is a technique of hypnosis. We often hear of the marvelous meditation practices of the Far East which enable the practitioners to control the heart rate, lower the body temperature or survive some unusual ordeal. Transcendental meditation also enables people to feel healthier and more at ease. Any technique which relaxes the conscious mind sufficiently will enable the unconscious mind to employ its resources in improving mental and physical health.

Hypnotherapists employ many different methods to facilitate this communication with the unconscious mind. Whatever technique is used, the prime objective is to relax the conscious mind so that it will not interfere with the natural responses of the unconscious. The more involved the subject becomes in the process of relaxation, the easier the responses to suggestion.

It should be emphasized that some people have great difficulty in relinquishing voluntary control of their minds and cannot become deeply involved in the hypnotic process. They may feel that they have not been influenced by suggestions in any way. It sometimes comes as a surprise to these people that the unconscious mind is taking some heed of the suggestions and eventually makes appropriate and effective responses.

Hypnoanalysis

I have found that certain important steps must be completed for effective hypnoanalysis to occur.

1. Location of the first critical experience

Once the appropriate communication has been established with the unconscious mind, the first step is to discover the patient's initial critical experience. The unconscious mind must be directed to locate the very first event which evoked feelings of guilt, shame or embarrassment. Prior to the advent of hypnotherapy, this approach was virtually impossible because the experience was so rarely accessible to the conscious memory, particularly when the first critical event was natal or pre-natal.

This earliest critical experience is usually associated with uncomfortable feelings, some of which the patient may become aware of for the first time. Occasionally the experience is so discomforting that perception of it is extremely limited. However, a frightening or painful feeling must be faced with courage. The unconscious mind has located this experience by the simple process of tracing the uncomfortable feeling to its source.

The patient may or may not be able to determine the details of this experience at a conscious level. Apart from satisfying his curiosity, his detailed conscious knowledge of the actual circumstances is not necessary for the next essential step.

2. Identification of the repressed feeling

When the critical experience has been located, the repressed emotions—sadness, anger, fear or a combination of any or all of these feelings—will emerge. Sometimes the feeling has all the intensity of the original event, and it is very important to allow an experience to fully release its associated feelings. An intense feeling reaching conscious awareness is called an abreaction since it is a reaction from the original cause of tension, free from any repressive action.

3. Acceptance of the repressed emotion

The originally repressed emotion has been unfelt and has therefore not been accepted. This next important step in therapy is the acceptance of this repressed emotion. If the patient has been able to experience the emotion in its original intensity, he has also been able to admit it. It is an emotion that is rightfully his, and he need no longer be ashamed of it. This acceptance marks an important step forward in the release from prison. By accepting the emotion, he has dealt with the greatest fear that underlies the guilt feeling—the threat of abandonment.

Repressing an emotion does not cancel it. In fact, such a response will ensure that it persists long after the need for it has disappeared.

4. Recognition of the current irrelevance of the previously repressed emotion

Now that the patient has been able to accept the emotion, it is time to determine whether there is any further need to retain it. The emotion is only necessary if it serves to protect him from danger. In nearly every case the original danger has long since passed and the emotion that has resulted is no longer requisite for protection. The patient must apply his new understanding to determine whether he still needs that emotion. A strong effort is necessary to relinquish an emotion that has probably been active for many years below the level of consciousness.

5. Relinquishing the unnecessary emotion

Merely deciding that an emotion is no longer necessary may not be enough to dispel it. A new solution must be developed for the problem which was originally dealt with by the repression of the unacceptable emotion. This new solution will vary with the problem and the person dealing with it. Usually certain fixed ingredients are available for any such solution. First, there is a recognition that the problem no long provokes fear. The patient now has the resources to care for and protect himself. Second, he must recognize that the original threat of abandonment was probably never likely, for his parent cared more for him than he had originally believed. Third, he must understand that all human beings have a right to their feelings so long as they are properly controlled. Finally, the patient must recognize that he had done nothing in this particular critical experience to alienate himself permanently from other members of the human race.

The patient always attains a profound sense of peace at this stage. When he has found a satisfactory solution, he will develop a sense of self-acceptance and wholeness which he had previously lacked. He will be able to say that he is as good and as important as any other human being—and he will now feel that this is true.

If any part of the mind has difficulty accepting its essential "O.K.-ness," other critical experiences must be subjected to hypnoanalysis. They must be located and examined and the repressed emotion recognized, accepted and relinquished. Only when all repressed emotion has been freed will the patient be free. This phase of hypnoanalysis must be completed with care and thoroughness.

In stage 1 through hypnosis we have initially made contact with all the memories of events contained in the three ego states. In stage 2 the Child ego state yields repressed feelings. Any guilt we discover is caused by the Parent ego state, which reminds the Child ego state that the expression of certain emotions may bring about the real parent's disapproval. If the emotion at the recollection of this experience is intense, as in an abreaction, then the Parent ego state's repressive forces have failed. The patient's realization that the disaster forecast by the Parent does not follow is therapeutic in permanently freeing the previously repressed emotion.

In stage 3 indications that the repressed emotion has now been accepted usually follow Adult intervention on the Child's behalf, pleading to the Parent that this emotion is indeed permissible. The Adult has been able to persuade the Parent that he need no longer prevent the Child from expressing that feeling.

In stage 4 recognition of the current irrelevance of the previously repressed emotion follows the Adult reasoning with the Child that things have now changed, that he is grown up. He can deal with the problem in a more mature manner so that the particular emotion which no longer serves a useful purpose can be discarded. Stage 5 may required all of the ingenuity of the Adult ego state to find a means to give up an outdated emotion. This stage is very important.

Whatever means the Adult ego state finds, it must be acceptable to both the Parent and the Child and must be utilized by them before the conflict over this particular issue comes to an end. At this juncture hypnoanalysis proper is also completed.

Throughout the hypnoanalytical procedure, the fundamental assumption maintains that the Adult ego state can find a solution underlying the Parent/Child conflict provided it is given sufficient information. The hypnotherapist must skillfully use these techniques to pry such information from the unconscious memories of the Parent and the Child. He must also persuade both the Child and the Parent that the resolution of their conflict is in their mutual best interest.

Chapter Eleven

The Prisoner

The prisoner in his cell spends long hours brooding over his past and dreaming about freedom. But the grey walls and the prison bars bring him back to reality before his fantasies afford him any relief.

Once he tried to escape. He laid elaborate schemes for eluding the guards and slipping through the door to freedom, but he was unsuccessful. The guards were not fooled by his ruses, and the chains that bound him withstood his assaults. Now with all hope gone, his sentence seems to stretch on endlessly ahead of him.

If you feel like this prisoner, you are fully aware that the only way to leave prison forever is to gain a complete pardon. All other escapes provide but a temporary release. A full pardon involves a reassessment of the crime for which you have been imprisoned. The evidence for conviction must be reheard, and all of the arguments against your imprisonment must be vigorously presented by a well-informed advocate. Hypnotherapy is an excellent means by which this may be accomplished.

If you are not certain whether your mind is imprisoned, carefully review the case histories already described. Persons who suffer from psychosomatic disorders are imprisoned. Anyone who is stricken by inexplicable anxieties and depressions, phobias or any of the physical disorders which are known to have an emotional origin or component is also imprisoned. Medical practitioners today acknowledge an important emotional component in the cause of such illnesses as heart disease, arthritis, hypertension and even cancer.

It is fairly obvious that anyone suffering from a drug addiction is imprisoned. The addiction itself is an additional chain that restricts and binds the sufferer. Anyone who is unable to function satisfactorily in normal, social or sexual settings is a mental prisoner. In each of these circumstances the mind is imprisoned by an idea which cripples and prevents it from functioning freely.

You may have recognized yourself in one of these categories, but perhaps you are still not sure. How can you determine whether or not you are imprisoned? Ask yourself, "Do I feel free? Am I able to express my full potential? Do I feel content with the person that I am? Do I like myself?"

If you can answer "Yes" to all of these questions, you enjoy great freedom. I trust that this book will enable you to direct others who are not so fortunate.

Should you recognize yourself as a prisoner, however, you need to act. The escapes that you have read about have been engineered with the aid of hypnosis. I believe that anyone who wants to break free should seek the help of a reputable hypnotherapist, who will help him discover those experiences which have led him to lock up a part of his feeling mind so that he now functions well below his potential.

Unfortunately, very few people have access to a skilled hypnotherapist or to any therapist who can help them in this way. All is not lost, however. You can do a great deal for yourself to locate your prison and identify the means of escape.

In each of us there is an impartial part of the personality which assesses information and experience in a rational, non-judgmental fashion. Our Adult ego state is continuously gathering new information about the world we live in. This ego state recognizes inconsistencies in our views and helps us to make intelligent, reasonable decisions.

Some of the life decisions we base our present views upon were made long before this part of us was in possession of the vast amount of information it now possesses. Whenever it is called upon to do so, our Adult can render an updated opinion on an old decision. It can always help us revise a decision that has resulted in mental imprisonment.

Self-Worth

Do you feel that you are as good and as important as every other human being? If you are a mental prisoner, you probably do not feel that good. At times you may feel like an intruder, an outsider—no sense of belonging, no secure habitation.

Yet you know that this cannot be true. You are a human being and have as much right on this planet as anyone else. Perhaps you lack some physical attributes enjoyed by others, but you can readily see that all human beings have some imperfections. You may not be as gifted as some of your friends, but neither are you as dull or uninformed as others.

Despite the fact that you "know" you are as good and as important as others, you are unable to feel that way. Why? Because you have been imprisoned for a crime resulting from your experiences, and your Parent ego state is constantly summoning up your guilt, which prevents you from feeling as good as you have a right to feel.

There is no denying that you once acted in a way that was unacceptable to someone close to you, or you vented a feeling that could not be admitted. But was that really a crime? Even if it were, must you continue to punish yourself after these many years? Guilt ensues when you lock up a part of your mind so effectively that it cannot accept your proper worth. You would like to heed your Adult, which gives assurance that you are just as good as anyone else, but guilt feelings interfere. Until you can find out why you still feel guilty, you cannot accept the liberated feeling of being a worthwhile human being.

How can you reach the source of the problem? Hypnosis can best help us obtain the information we seek. Even light hypnosis is extremely effective in this respect, and since ninety-five percent of the population can enter this state, hypnoanalytical techniques can be used with the majority of mental prisoners.

Before we examine how to do this, however, let us look more closely at the face of the prisoner.

The Face of the Prisoner

The troubled prisoner usually turns to a physician or some other counselor for help. But the emotional element of his problem may be so well concealed that it escapes the detection of the most astute observer.

1. The Psychosomatic Disorders

All psychosomatic disorders are by definition the result of mental imprisonment. The list of illnesses which can be termed psychosomatic grows longer every day. Such disorders masquerade as purely physical illnesses but are directly related to emotional problems. Although all illnesses probably have an emotional component, this element is the precipitating factor in psychosomatic illness.

Migraine and Tension Headaches

Along with tension headaches, migraine is the commonest problem for which the help of hypnotherapy is sought. Migraine is believed to result from the effects of tension upon the blood vessels of the head. This tension initially causes the vessels to contract, but relaxation at a later time allows them to dilate, causing the typical pain. When the muscles of the head rather than the blood vessels contract, tension headaches result.

Conventional therapy is restricted to administering rest or drugs for the relief of pain and tension. Ergot and its derivatives are used specifically for migraine because of their ability to contract the painfully dilated blood vessels, relieving the pressure from tender nerve endings in the head. By contrast, direct suggestion in hypnosis stimulates the healing powers of the unconscious mind. These powers can duplicate any of the useful effects of drugs without causing side effects.

Physicians recognize that treating a migraine headache after it has become established is much like closing the stable door after the horse has bolted. They attempt to prevent attacks by counseling the patient to avoid conflicts which create tension, or they prescribe drugs which keep the patient relaxed. The analytical hypnotherapist recognizes that the tension which precipitates migraine is present for a good reason, even though that reason is probably out of date and out of step with the patient's present adult life. The victim is unaware of the emotional trap in which he is imprisoned. Only when he has unlocked his mind can he be free from the headaches.

All analytical hypnotherapy patients are taught self-hypnosis so that they may use autosuggestion during an attack to relieve pain. However, we do not feel that therapy is totally successful until the migraine sufferer is completely free of headaches. The patient can then use his self-hypnosis to get in touch with his own vast unconscious resources for other useful purposes.

Migraine sufferers are usually trapped in the prison of anger. They stubbornly retain old repressed anger about which they still feel guilty. Whenever they find themselves in a situation in which they experience normal human anger, it too is repressed with guilt. The resulting tension causes the initial contraction of the blood vessels of the head, and migraine naturally follows.

Rarely do migraine sufferers realize the poverty of their lives until they resolve their tensions. Suddenly they begin to experience a joy in living that they had not previously known, including an increased sense of self-confidence and well-being.

Asthma

Asthma is generally considered an allergic condition. The bronchial tubes of the asthmatic, responding in an overly sensitive manner to substances in the air, contract so strongly on meeting these substances that they block the sufferer's flow of air, making breathing difficult. The noxious substance is effectively kept out, but so is vital oxygen. Asthma is a classic example of a protective response which has become harmful.

Although asthma is considered to be primarily of allergic origin and thus may be controlled by drugs, I include it here because attacks of asthma can be precipitated by purely emotional factors. In fact, almost any allergic response can be reproduced by purely emotional factors, and all allergic illnesses may be associated with a more or less significant emotional element.

Unfortunately, the asthma sufferer is usually unaware of the existence of any emotional problem. He is frequently misled into restricting his search for the cause to allergic factors where few or none really exist.

When the significance of the emotional factors has been recognized, doctors warn patients to avoid conflicts and prescribe sedatives or tranquilizers. This approach is sometimes effective but is rarely completely satisfactory.

Analytical hypnotherapy enables the asthma sufferer to locate the emotional causes of his asthma so that he can deal with them in an appropriate way. Meanwhile, the asthma sufferer can be taught to use self-hypnosis to control the spasm of the bronchial tubes during attacks.

The asthmatic is trapped in a prison of pain and sadness. He is not allowed to feel his hurt. He is unable to cry, for his bronchial tubes are holding back his tears by their contractions. Any situation resembling that in which he unconsciously feels hurt or rejection may precipitate this repressive mechanism.

Peptic Ulcer

Stomach and duodenal ulcers strike nervous individuals. All of us have experienced "butterflies in the stomach," and we all have been aware of tension in the abdomen. Some people will even vomit or have diarrhea when they are emotionally disturbed. Therefore it is easy to understand how stomach ulcers occur in those who are constantly tense.

The usual therapy for peptic ulcers consists in the administration of medicines and a diet which reduces the acid content of the stomach. Tension-reducing tranquilizers are also frequently administered. Ulcer sufferers are advised to avoid conflict.

Direct suggestion in hypnosis can often duplicate the accomplishment of drugs. Analytical hypnotherapy patients additionally benefit from learning to use self-hypnosis for these effects, while simultaneously discovering the source of the tension responsible for their stomach disorder. Most of these patients are locked in the prison

103

of anger.

Colitis

There are many names for the different disturbances of the bowel in which recurrent diarrhea, constipation and abdominal pain are present. Some of these have a definite organic basis, but the majority can properly be considered psychosomatic. Such cases will probably respond temporarily to the relaxing effect of direct suggestion in hypnosis, but successful hypnoanalysis will produce more permanent results.

When the patient is freed from his prison—likely one of fear—he is once again able to have normal bowel function without discomfort and can dispense with the drugs which have previously played such an important part in his therapy.

Cardiovascular Diseases

The greatest killers in modern times are the cardiovascular diseases, including diseases of the heart and blood vessels. Some of these are due to infection or to some structural or congential deformity, but the majority are, at least in part, psychosomatic.

A certain type of personality, distinguished by his attitude toward life, is most susceptible to high blood pressure and heart problems. He is likely to be a hard driving, ambitious individual. High blood pressure, normally occasioned by extreme tension, is physiologically achieved when the heart works extra hard and the blood vessels contract so that it is harder for the blood to flow throughout the body. When increased blood, flowing to certain organs, is urgently required for extreme physical exertion, this is a normal response, but it is certainly unnecessary for the business man sitting in his office. Although he does not need raised blood pressure, his body works extra hard in direct response to the same suppressed emotion which makes him ambitious and intense. He is likely to have excessive cholesterol in his blood, which will cause his blood vessels to harden prematurely and become constricted, with a tendency to block up. Blockage of the blood vessels in the heart will cause a heart attack.

Hypnosis can lower the blood pressure and slow the heart rate. It acts upon the nervous system through its communication with the unconscious mind. These effects, though useful, tend to be temporary in the patient who is a candidate for cardiovascular disease. He must alter his attitude towards himself for more permanent results. In order to do this, he must first escape from the prison in which he is trapped. The commonest prison is that of guilt. Such a person does not feel that he has the right to exist. He must constantly prove that he should have the privilege of life.

Analytical hypnotherapy will help such a person to accept himself and allow him to relax and enjoy his existence as a normal human being. When he has accomplished this, he can permit his blood pressure to return to normal and his heart to slow down since the need to drive himself will have vanished.

Skin Diseases

Some skin diseases result from external irritation. Scabies is caused by a small parasite which invades the skin. Certain allergic skin disorders are brought about by the skin's oversensitivity to a mild irritant. In most cases the patient aggravates the damage by scratching the itch.

Other skin disorders are caused by internal disturbances. These skin disorders are psychosomatic, and doctors usually treat them with soothing applications or tranquilizers.

Hypnotherapy will help these skin conditions when direct suggestion is used. However, this approach will rarely be permanently effective until the reasons for the underlying tension have been dealt with.

Hypnoanalysis frequently enables skin disease sufferers to escape from their prison of anger from which their repressed hostility directed at the self, is usually expressed through scratching.

Menstrual Problems

Many readers may be surprised that I have listed menstrual disorders among the psychosomatic diseases, but in a great number of cases no organic cause can be found for painful conditions of irregular, excessive or absent menstruation.

Hypnosis can be used to correct these disorders by the simple method of giving direct suggestions. The improvement will be temporary when the underlying emotional problem persists, but analytical hypnotherapy can resolve these problems, which often are due to self-rejection and incarceration in the prison of guilt.

Sexual Dysfunction

In women sexual dysfunction includes frigidity, failure to achieve an orgasm and pain during intercourse. The latter might be so severe as to cause a spasm of the vagina, called vaginismus, which prevents normal sexual intercourse.

In men sexual dysfunction includes failure to achieve or maintain an erection, premature ejaculation or failure to ejaculate.

Almost invariably sexual dysfunction is the result of guilt; hypnotherapy offers the best hope of release from this prison.

2. The Habit Disorders

Compulsive behavior creates a great range of problems harmful to the individual. Bedwetting, nail biting and thumb sucking are compulsive activities which are not serious but become the source of discomfort.

Other habits pose a real health hazard, yet compulsives often resist every effort to end them. Excessive smoking, drug addiction and alcoholism are the most common examples. Victims may recognize the consequences of their habits and yet be powerless to forego them, for the habit serves a purpose so vital to unconscious emotional needs that the attainment of good physical health remains secondary. I have seen patients whose smoking had caused severe heart disease, whose alcoholism had damaged their livers, and whose drug taking had brought them within inches of death persist in these habits in a compulsive manner.

Why should this be so? All of these unfortunate people are locked in a prison of pain and sadness. Not permitted to accept these repressed feelings, they can only experience them at a deeply unconscious level and keep them from consciousness by means of the devices which form the bad habit. They have been condemned to their habit as their means of tolerating life, even if such behavior shortens life or renders it extremely uncomfortable.

By locating the critical experiences causing unconscious pain and sadness and by allowing acceptance of that pain, analytical hypnotherapy can permit patients to escape to freedom from their prison. The drugs, the cigarettes, the alcohol used to repress the pain are no longer required.

Obesity

Obesity is such an extremely common problem that I am treating it separately. It mixes features of a psychosomatic as well as a habit disorder.

As a general physician I have treated many people for obesity, using all kinds of diet programs, medications, and exhortations. I have bullied, cajoled, used injections and made direct hypnotic suggestions. Many patients have initially lost weight quite well, and some have even reached their target weight, but sad to say, nearly all of them regained their previous weight and sometimes even more after a year or two.

Since I have confined my practice to a purely hypnoanalytical approach, I have finally realized why the obese experience such difficulty in losing weight and staying slim. Almost every obese patient is unconsciously afraid to be slim and is deliberately eating in order to remain fat! Such people may consciously stay on a diet for a while, but when they start to lose weight, the fear of being thin becomes so strong that they are impeled to eat and put the weight back on again. At a conscious level, of course, they are only aware of another failure. So long as this fear of becoming thin persists, they are doomed to failure.

Most obese people expect the hypnotherapist to cure them by giving their unconscious mind a suggestion not to eat. In my experience this approach has never worked. A post-hypnotic suggestion of this kind rarely persists for any length of time simply because it will not be acceptable to the unconscious mind of the obese patient until the fear of becoming slim has been confronted.

Why are the obese afraid to become slim? They have learned to use their fat as a protection from the danger of expressing a forbidden feeling. Without the fat they will be exposed to the imagined dangers that the revealed feeling will incur. The fat is the physical expression of the mental walls that imprison the mind. In a small proportion of cases of obesity food is strongly associated with comfort and is used to assuage unconscious feelings of rejection and deprivation. In these cases such feelings must be recognized and relinquished if a successful reduction to a reasonable eating pattern is to be established.

When the patient is free to feel his previously concealed emotions, he no longer has the compulsion to overeat. At the same time, he may lose the driving need to shed weight which threw him into the seesaw of weight changes over the years. He will usually accept a new and more sensible pattern of eating, gradually and perhaps imperceptibly losing weight. One day a slimmer individual will recognize that he need not be anxious about his dieting.

3. The Emotional Disorders

This third group of prisoners is extremely important. Depression, anxieties, phobias and obsessions are some of the emotional disorders responsible for an immense amount of human misery.

Depressions

Those of us who have suffered from a deep depression know how trapped one feels within it. There seems to be no escape, no hope, no future. Nothing seems to be of value or importance, and only a sense of duty keeps one going. For some very depressed people even this becomes inadequate to provide them with sufficient motivation to carry on, and thus they experience a strong temptation to drop out of life altogether.

The depressed patient is suffering from a strong parental rejection. He has probably attempted to excel and may have succeeded, but whenever he fails, he finds himself face to face with his self-rejection and once again believes that he has no right to be. He is bad, unloved and unlovable. He knew this in the beginning, and despite all of his efforts, nothing has changed.

Analytical hypnotherapy gives the depressed patient the opportunity to reexamine his original assumptions about himself. He has the chance to apply to himself some of the wisdom that he would offer a colleague or a friend. He can see himself as he really is and recognize the need to break out of his burdensome prison for good. Hypnoanalysis does this by locating and dealing with the parental rejection which lies at the source of all depressions.

When the depression sufferer is able to get in touch with the real pain which his defenses have successfully concealed from him, he is at last able to relinquish it and accept himself despite his parent's rejection. He is at last free.

Anxiety

All of us experience fear at some time, but the anxiety sufferer is in an almost constant state of fear. He is walled in by his problem. He worries about everything—yesterday, today, tomorrow. Whatever you can name he has worried to death long ago. This constant state of anxiety may be associated with specific phobias which have their own particular brand of paralyzing anxiety. The sufferer from anxiety is always tense and reflects many of the symptoms that are popularly associated with tension. He will often respond surprisingly well to direct suggestions for relaxation given in hypnosis, which attests to the power of the unconscious mind. Such relief is usually short-lived, however, unless the true cause of the anxiety is discovered and dealt with permanently.

The victim of anxiety is obviously living in a prison of fear—in dread of fear itself. When he is brought face to face with the true cause of his fear, his mind is capable of handling the pressure once he has allowed himself to be really afraid. He now recognizes that he has a right to be afraid—as well as a right to relinquish that fear once it has served its purpose. At last he can accept the idea that he no longer needs it. It is outdated and totally irrelevant to the present.

Phobias

Most of those who suffer from a phobia do not talk about it. Ashamed of their problem, they dread the possibility of having their weakness exposed in public. They may fear elevators, airplanes, certain animals, spaces, heights, etc. The list goes on and on. How did it originate?

Most probably an extremely frightening experience happened which made the patient feel very guilty—so guilty that he was no longer able to feel his fear. Certain events precipitate his fear in the most intense manner, yet the intensity of the phobia prevents him from knowing and feeling the original fear about which he experiences so much guilt.

Although the phobic victim is extremely afraid, he is never consciously aware of his original fear, which is repressed by guilt and the phobia. In hypnoanalysis he can uncover the critical experiences and the guilt associated with them. When the phobia is no longer necessary, the subject will know his true fear and no longer feel guilty about it.

Obsessions

Obsessive or compulsive behavior is again a protective device to repress the knowledge of something about which the patient feels guilty. Once he can let himself know about it, he can make progress towards not feeling guilty and eventually control his compulsive behavior.

Much of our discussion of the different problems that a hypnotherapist sees in his practice may make the solution appear very simple. In reality, solutions *are* often simple. The greatest difficulty lies in discovering the solution and knowing how to apply it.

Chapter Twelve

Manufacturing The Key—
Self-Hypnosis

Although one can more easily learn hypnosis from an expert rather than from the mute pages of a book, it is unlikely that more than a small proportion of the readers of this book will have ready access to such an expert. I am therefore going to detail a procedure which I have found successful in enabling most people to reach a light or medium stage of hypnosis adequate for the analytical procedures which follow.

1. Physical Relaxation

The first step is to bring yourself to a state of complete physical relaxation. Some people will find this easy to accomplish while others need to practice repeatedly. Do not become discouraged if you do not immediately succeed.

Seat yourself in a comfortable chair at a time when you will be undisturbed for a while—at least a half hour. It is really important that you are physically comfortable and that nothing is going on which will distract you from devoting your maximum attention to self-hypnosis.

(a) Deep Breathing

When you are comfortable, take a long, very deep breath, hold it for a few seconds, and then let it out very slowly. If you are, or have been, a smoker, you will probably recognize that this is exactly what you do when you are tense and inhale on a cigarette. You may be surprised to find that this deep breath is just as relaxing without tobacco smoke.

Repeat the long, deep breath, hold it, and then let it out slowly. As you do, allow your whole body to sink deeply into the chair until you feel literally glued to the chair by your weight. Already you will have achieved a great deal of physical relaxation.

Now take a third long, deep breath and feel that relaxation spreading to every area of your body. If your eyes are not already shut, then let them close as your breath flows from your chest. Enjoy this beautiful relaxation for a few moments.

(b) Eyelid Relaxation

When you are ready, turn your attention to your eyelids and concentrate on the feeling in them. They may already be so heavy and relaxed that you do not want to open them. Imagine that they are so heavy that they will not open. Try to remember the feeling your eyes have when someone wants to awaken you from a lovely, deep sleep. They now feel so heavy that they simply do not want to open. Wait until you are certain that they are so relaxed that they cannot open before you test them. You will find that you have used your imagination so well that they will remain closed until you direct them otherwise.

Once you have tested your eyes and have found that they will not open, you know that your unconscious imagination has taken charge and you have allowed your conscious mind to relinquish its usual control.

(c) Body Relaxation

The next step is to spread that relaxation in your eyes and eyelids all the way through your body just like a blanket of relaxation from the top of your head down to the tips of your toes. You can completely relax your entire body. None of the muscles will have any desire to move at all. Enjoy that beautiful relaxation for as long as you wish. At first you may find that one or two minutes will be sufficient. At the end of this period tell yourself that when you count silently and slowly from one to five, your imagination will allow your eyes to open when you reach five and that when they do, you will feel really great—better than you have felt for a long time. Then count to five silently; your eyes will open and you will feel very good.

Do not progress beyond this stage until you have practiced it several times and feel proficient at it. Even if you never progress beyond this stage, you will have learned how to relax your body quickly and easily. This degree of relaxation can be used to relieve the minor tensions and anxieties which are frequently associated with all kinds of stressful circumstances. You will never regret having learned this relaxation technique. It is the first essential step in modern hypnosis.

If you experience any difficulty in persuading your eyes to stay closed, imagine that they are weighed down by heavy lead shutters—so heavy that they simply cannot be lifted. You might find it helpful to imagine that a layer of glue between the lids has stuck them firmly together. Remember, you have a responsive unconscious imagination. If all else fails, pretend that the eyelids cannot open; so long as you keep up this pretense, they will remain closed.

In this simple exercise you have amply demonstrated that your unconscious mind and imagination can be given control of your body and that it can be asked to return that control on short notice. By relaxing conscious control, you have made a big step forward to freeing your unconscious imagination.

2. Mental Relaxation

Only when you are certain that you have mastered the first step of physical relaxation and can produce it at will should you proceed to the second stage of self-hypnosis, mental relaxation. Whether the first stage has taken you several minutes or several days to master does not matter. You will only benefit from the second stage when you have mastered the first, so do not act in haste. When you return once again to the physically relaxed stage, you will be ready to enter the second stage—relaxation of the mind which will complement the tranquility of the body.

Imagine yourself looking at a blackboard on which all of the numbers from fifty down to one are written. When you can imagine them clearly, rub the number fifty off the blackboard so completely that it has gone completely out of your mind. Proceed to the next number. Erase that from your imaginary blackboard before continuing, making sure that it too has vanished from your mind and has completely disappeared. Continue with this process, erasing all the numbers completely. During the process you will find that you are becoming more relaxed mentally as each number fades. You will soon feel so mentally tired that you will want to erase all of the remaining numbers off the blackboard at once. Now you have a completely blank blackboard and a very relaxed mind—so relaxed that you are ready for the third stage, which will use your imagination to its full capacity. Bring the numbers back and count silently from one to five as before; you will be wide awake, feeling even better than you did previously.

Before you proceed to the third stage, practice what you have already learned at least three times so that you can produce mental relaxation as often as you wish.

3. Imagery

In the third stage, the production of imagery, you will receive an indication of your ability to use self-hypnosis. In this stage suggestions are accepted by the imagination. The positive suggestions that you will learn to give yourself will receive maximum unconscious attention.

Return once again to stage two. When you have made your mind totally blank, picture yourself in a pleasant place doing something that you really like. If you have chosen a waterside scene, see the water clearly. Note whether it is smooth or wavy. If it is wavy, hear the sounds of the waves, whether quiet or rather loud. If the sun is shining, feel the warmth of the sun. If it gets too hot, feel yourself move into the shade. Since it is your picture, be totally comfortable in it. Look around; if anyone else is there, note what they are doing. Pay attention to every sound, feeling or smell that you notice. Enjoy it. Once again, when you have reveled in the scene as much as you need to, count back from one to five and you will be wide awake but perhaps amazed at the vividness of all you have seen and experienced.

You have now learned all that you need to know about entering self-hypnosis. You will gain great benefit by giving yourself positive suggestions when you are in this relaxed state. Tell yourself that you will feel cheerful, relaxed, self-confident and energetic when you awaken. You will soon be surprised how effective these suggestions prove to be. This feature has been known for centuries and used in many guises. It is effective because your unconscious mind is listening carefully in hypnosis, accepting suggestions and acting upon them.

This third stage of this program of self hypnosis is probably the most powerful. It is also the stage in which post hypnotic suggestions are most likely to be effective. You are therefore to be encouraged to practice until you are proficient at reaching and using this stage of self hypnosis.

Much of the history of the success of hypnosis has been due to the effectiveness of suggestions given in this highly receptive stage of unconscious imagery. By incorporating images of the person that you would wish to become and imagining yourself behaving in a positive manner in situations in which you were previously negative, these images will have a potent posthypnotic effect whose power will sometimes surprise you. For example should you have a problem with overeating, by simply visualizing yourself as slim and seeing yourself being satisfied by non-fattening foods will have a strong posthypnotic effect.

Certainly suggestions of wellbeing, confidence, relaxation and freedom from discomfort can always be emphasized by appropriate imagery involving these suggestions.

It may well be that this limited use of self hypnosis will meet all of your present therapeutic needs and that analysis is not required in your case. Nevertheless I would urge you not to forgo the ego strengthening and assertiveness training programs detailed at the end of the following chapter on self analysis.

If you are a prisoner of the mind, it is highly probable that these suggestions will not be as effective as they could be. They may only be temporarily successful because a part of your unconscious mind rejects them. This is why hypnotherapy using only direct suggestion is less effective than analytical hypnotherapy, which is directed at removing any objection to the acceptance of a direct suggestion.

If you are not a prisoner of the mind, you will be able to adopt any of the positive suggestions that you choose to give yourself. Experiment with the simple suggestions I have already outlined before progressing to more complex ones, such as those for the relief of pain and the development of anesthesia.

I am concerned here with the prisoner of the mind and his need to be free. In the next chapter I will examine self-hypnosis as a channel of communication with the unconscious mind. By yourself you can turn the key in the lock of your prison and free yourself from the bonds of guilt.

Chapter Thirteen

Turning The Key Yourself

You have learned to relax your conscious mind sufficiently to allow useful suggestions to reach your unconscious mind. You have put its great resources to work in translating thought into action, practicing until you have become proficient. Now you are ready for the most important stage—self-analysis, using hypnosis.

Establishing Unconscious Signaling

In order to locate unconscious memories as an analytical hypnotherapist would, you will need to establish a signaling system which your unconscious mind can use in order to communicate with you at a conscious level. We know that unconscious movements are related to unconscious ideas. If we can set up an unconscious movement which indicates the unconscious idea "yes," and another which signals the unconscious idea "no," we will establish an excellent channel of communication.

The procedure for establishing this signaling is simple but requires a little patience. Read the following instructions several times carefully before attempting to carry them out.

Return once again to the deep relaxed state in which you were able to blank your mind and accept images. Then start to think "yes," "yes," "yes" over and over again until you feel the need to let your head nod in agreement. When this happens, ask your inner mind to raise one of your fingers on your dominant hand as a signal for "yes." You may have to wait for this to occur, but meanwhile continue to think "yes" repeatedly. Eventually one of the fingers on your dominant hand will begin to feel light and will slowly jerk upward as your unconscious mind allows the idea of "yes" to flow into it. Note which finger that is, because from now on you will think of it as your "yes" finger.

Repeat this process, but this time think "no" continuously until your head begins to feel like shaking "no" and another finger on the same hand begins to feel light and lifts. This is your "no" finger. Make a mental note of it.

At times you may ask your unconscious mind a question, but for reasons of its own it does not want to answer. You need a signal to let you know this. Repeat the above process once again, but this time keep thinking, "I don't want to answer," "I don't want to answer." Meanwhile ask your unconscious mind to select another finger. You have now established your signaling system and are ready for analysis.

Using the Signals

Now that your unconscious mind possesses a set of signals which it can use to respond to your questions, you can obtain admittance to information which had previously been inaccessible to you at a conscious level. Each time you wish to question your unconscious mind, return to the relaxed state.

First, ask your unconscious mind some general questions in order to get used to this signaling system. Your first question should be, "Is it all right for me to ask questions about my problem?" In most cases the answer will be "yes," and you have made a good start toward analysis. However, if the answer is "no," you have a problem. Ask the question again to make sure. If the answer is still "no," you will not secure the cooperation of your unconscious mind on your own and will have to seek the aid of a hypnotherapist.

Let us assume that you gain an affirmative answer to the question, "Is it all right to ask questions?" Proceed to the next question, which will establish further unconscious cooperation. Pick the symptom which concerns you most and ask, "Is my symptom due to an emotional problem?" Again you should get a "yes" answer before proceeding.

Next inquire, "Is it all right for me to know the cause of this emotional problem?" Await a positive response before proceeding. You are now ready for the first step in self-analysis using hypnosis. Allow yourself a full hour for this process. You may not need it, but since you will not know beforehand, it is best to provide plenty of time.

SELF-ANALYSIS
1. The Location of the Critical Experience

The first stage in any analysis is the identification of the critical experience during which the crisis responsible for the emotional problem occurred. This is the time at which the crime liable for the imprisonment was committed. It is the experience which made you feel guilty, producing the constraints which have bound you ever since.

It is important that you follow these directions in faithful detail in order to be completely successful. But it is not necessary to complete

118

the whole stage at any one time.

a) **The review of all unconscious tensions:** Ask your unconscious mind to review all of your old, outdated unconscious tensions and to indicate when this has been accomplished by lifting the "yes" finger.

b) **Location of the earliest tension:** Ask your unconscious mind to determine the earliest of these tensions and to indicate when this has been accomplished by once again raising the "yes" finger.

c) **Review of the earliest tension:** Ask your unconscious mind to review this earliest tension and the experience responsible for it in complete detail and to let you know when this has been done by raising the "yes" finger.

d) **Elevation of the unconscious memory to consciousness:** First of all, ask your unconscious mind if it is all right for you to know about the experience which is responsible for your problem and, if so, to indicate by a "yes" signal. If you receive an affirmative response, direct your unconscious mind to bring the memory of this experience to a level where you can remember it consciously.

At this stage of the analysis you may well begin to feel unusual emotions which are often unclear at first. They will later amalgamate into a specific feeling which is likely to be quite uncomfortable. The experience causing this feeling will at first be fragmentary but will soon become more clearly defined. The feelings that accompany it may be those of desolation, sadness, anger or fear. Whatever the feelings may be, do not yield to the temptation to block them off. With perseverance you will eventually know all of the experience which has been responsible for the feelings. If this does not occur and the critical circumstance still remains hidden, repeat the above steps as described.

In my experience the uncovering of the previously repressed emotion may in itself be followed by intense relief. Should this be so, it is because you have unconsciously progressed through the stages of acceptance of the forbidden and repressed emotion to the stage of discarding it. You may have even resolved the problem originally causing it. In any case, the succeeding steps should be followed in strict sequence but can be postponed to your next analytical session.

2. Review and Acceptance of the Previously Repressed Emotion

You have succeeded in locating the critical experience and the previously concealed emotion associated with it. Your next task is to gain unconscious acceptance of this emotion. To do this, simply ask your unconscious mind to use all of your unconscious wisdom, understanding and compassion to look at and review all of the now visible experience, indicating when this has been accomplished by lifting the "yes" finger.

3. Recognition of the Present Irrelevance of the Previously Repressed Emotion

The time has come for you to use your unconscious mind to discover whether you now have any further need for the old emotion which had been repressed.

To do this, ask your unconscious mind, "With the understanding I now possess, must I preserve that old tension?" You should receive a "no" to this question before proceeding with the next step. If you do not, once again ask your unconscious mind to review the experience, using all of your unconscious wisdom. When this has been done once again, inquire whether you still need to keep that old and outdated emotion. You will probably now obtain the "no" that you are seeking.

If, on the other hand, you still receive a "yes," settle for that at this time since there may still be a need for some of the old emotion. Instead now ask, "Do I still need ALL of that outdated emotion?" If you get a "no" to this question, it is clear that your unconscious mind is not prepared to release all of the emotion at present, and it may be that you are consciously aware of the reason for this.

4. Relinquishing the Unnecessary Outdated Tension

You have now decided that you no longer need some or all of the outdated emotion, and you need to find a satisfactory means of relinquishing the unnecessary tension. Once again, call upon the resources of your unconscious mind to find a way to let the old outdated emotion go. Simply ask, "Using all of my unconscious understanding and wisdom, please find a way in which this old, useless and outdated tension can be released, and indicate when this way has been found by raising the 'yes' finger."

When that finger lifts, you may or may not be consciously aware of the appropriate solution that has been discovered by your unconscious mind, but you will already begin to feel a lessening of tension.

5. Resolution of the Outdated Tension

You are ready to surrender the old tension. Ask your unconscious mind to supply the solution it has found by the use of your unconscious wisdom to the part of your mind that has had to deal with the problem creating the tension. Ask for a signal when that solution has been accepted and the tension at last completely relinquished.

When the solution has been put into effect and you have given up the old tension, you will feel a great sense of relief. Await the signal confirming the complete resolution of the tension before proceeding to the final step.

6. Rehabilitation

It is one thing to find a solution to a problem, another to have it working in practice. With hypnosis the actual working conditions can be imagined quite faithfully. To do this, simply instruct your unconscious mind to imagine the solution that has been accepted, being applied in three different relevant problematic situations, and to signal when this has been accomplished.

You may have been able to complete all of these stages in one session. Whether or not this is possible, it is time to take a rest. You have done well. Reinforce your general well-being by direct suggestions and return to the remainder of your self-analysis as soon as you again have sufficient time to devote to it.

During the procedure you may have been aware of each line of thought that your unconscious mind has pursued. It is quite likely, however, that much has remained unconscious.

If you have not been successful in completing all of these stages, do not be downhearted. Give yourself direct suggestions that you will be successful and try once again after a rest from the analysis. If your progress remains disappointingly slow, you should renew your efforts to obtain expert hypnotherapeutic assistance.

Further Analysis

Having resolved a long standing problem, you will no doubt be feeling very good. It is probable, however, that you have other unconscious tensions which must be dealt with before you can enjoy the true relief of complete freedom.

How are you to know if further analysis should be pursued? A totally free human being, with a completely unlocked mind, believes that he is just as good as any other human being and feels convinced that this is so.

Ask your unconscious mind, "Does every part of my inner mind now feel and believe that I am just as good and important as any other human being, living or dead?" If the answer to this important question is an immediate "yes," then you are ready for the final stages of self-therapy. However, if a negative response arises, a part of your mind is still harboring a problem and you should continue analysis.

In order to proceed, ask your unconscious mind to review all of your unconscious memories and to stop at any experience which is preventing you from feeling as good and as important as any other human being. Ask that it verify its location of the experience by raising the "yes" finger. Deal with this experience in precisely the same way that you handled the first one, following each of the six steps outlined. You may find that it will not take as long to resolve this problem, for your unconscious mind now knows exactly what is required of it. You should have no difficulty in completing your work with it in one session.

Repeat the question about self-worth and deal with every experience which is preventing you from fully accepting yourself. Eventually you will have dealt with all of the experiences which have been responsible for your present tensions and will have resolved them satisfactorily.

Again let me reiterate that if you run into any difficulty whatsoever, you must seek expert hypnotherapeutic help.

Ego Strengthening

For most of your life your ego has taken a back seat, severely restricted by the problems you have now resolved. You will surely encounter many new challenges along life's stormy path, however, and you must be able to deal with them. Otherwise you will again seek refuge in the only secure place you have known—prison! You must develop in your ego sufficient strength to deal with these problems appropriately so that your new found freedom will be permanent.

No matter how self-confident you feel, it does no harm to repeat this ego strengthening procedure quite frequently.

First of all, ask your unconscious mind, "Does every part of my unconscious mind now believe that I am just as important and good as any other human being living or dead?" You should now receive a strong "yes" signal. In any case, ask your unconscious mind to repeat several times "I am just as good and important as any other human being living or dead." I believe that the recording of a powerful positive message like this tends to erase all of the other negative recordings that you have been carrying in your unconscious mind throughout your life.

Return to your deep relaxation and ask your unconscious mind the following questions:

1. Does my inner mind agree that I have the right to every one of

my normal human feelings, whether or not they are pleasant?

2. Does my inner mind agree that I have the right and the duty to respect and protect every one of my normal human feelings, whether they be pleasant or unpleasant?

3. Does my inner mind agree that I have the right to keep any of my normal human feelings as long as I need them and a right to let them go whenever they become unnecessary?

If each of these questions receives the appropriate affirmative response, proceed with the next question:

4. Do I need to feel guilty, ashamed or embarrassed by any of my normal human feelings? This question should now receive a strong "no" answer.

You may have obtained a negative reply to any one of the first three questions. If so, you must discover the reason in order for ego strengthening to be entirely successful.

You will need to ask questions which will enable you to identify which basic emotion is still unacceptable. For example, "Do I have a right to my normal human feelings of sadness?" Prescribe similar questions in order to identify your unconscious attitudes regarding the other emotions of happiness, anger, love, fear and security. When you have specified the feeling that troubles you still, utilize the analytical techniques you have learned to locate the experience involving the unacceptable emotion. You should be able to relinquish the outdated emotion and the guilt associated with it, thus resolving your inner conflict.

Return then to ego strengthening, obtaining a "yes" to all of the first three questions and a "no" to the fourth.

When this ego strengthening phase has been satisfactorily completed, you will be ready for the final phase of therapy—assertiveness training.

Assertiveness Training

For years you have considered yourself inferior to others and have behaved as if you were inferior. In reality, you are as worthy as others. It is essential that you overcome feelings of inferiority if your newfound freedom is to become permanent. You are in need of new guidelines to replace the old self-rejecting ones. This is why assertiveness training is so important. Incidentally, do not confuse assertiveness with aggressiveness. The free, assertive individual is never aggressive, although his self-confidence might be mistaken for aggressiveness by the casual observer.

Once again engage the techniques of self-hypnosis to communicate with your unconscious mind, which must be ready to undertake three important resolutions. Put them to your unconscious mind in the following manner:

1. "Will every part of my inner mind promise never to put any other part down?"

2. "Will every part of my inner mind promise never to allow anyone to put me down?"

3. "Will my inner mind promise never to allow me knowingly to put anyone else down?"

The phrase "put down" is usually understood quite well at an unconscious level. It refers to the discounting or devaluing of feelings and not to proper and just criticism. If you call yourself stupid or use some other derogatory name, you are putting yourself down. However, if you recognize that you have made a mistake, you are not demeaning yourself by being aware of it. You also disparage yourself when you discount your feelings and say such things as "I should not feel angry (hurt or afraid, etc.)." You have a right to your feelings; any time you discount them or allow someone else to do so, you are putting yourself down.

If you have received strong "yes" signals to these questions, this final part of therapy has been satisfactorily completed. Nevertheless, I would advise that you repeat the ego strengthening and the assertiveness training suggestions every day until you are certain that you can keep these three promises under all circumstances.

If you have come this far successfully with me, you will no doubt be aware of a tremendous increase in your feelings of well-being and self-confidence. Without any conscious effort you are beginning to stick up for yourself, and people who previously ignored your views and opinions now obviously respect you. Less concerned about others' opinions, you will remain interested in their views without sacrificing yours to theirs. Most of all, you will find yourself doing things with increased energy, acting because you want to and not because a certain response is expected of you.

Anyone who has been locked up in a mental prison most of his life will discover that this freedom is a wonderful experience. Some former patients will supply individual tales of escape to freedom.

Chapter Fourteen

Escape Stories

1. H.B.

I hated my life. I recognize now, of course, that I really hated myself. For more than forty years my life was a hopeless struggle. Trying to be better than I was, I had failed miserably. To my friends I apparently had everything anyone could wish for—three lovely daughters, a loving husband, no financial burdens. Yet I hated it all. Nothing seemed to be right.

I often asked myself, "Why does my loving husband care for me?" but I could never find an answer. I knew that I had always loved him, but I was never able to tell him so. I could never allow myself to show him the affection that I knew he truly deserved. Many times when I felt things go wrong, I simply hated and hated. I tried not to let my anger show, but it always smouldered within me, fixing my husband and my children at arm's length.

I always felt very tense—as if my insides were stretched as taut as a drum. My head seemed as if it was bursting. My sympathetic physician offered medication to help me relax, but I never took any medicine, for I had an intense fear of becoming dependent on drugs. The only time I did take a prescription, after desperate persuasion from my husband, I threw up and could hardly breathe. I simply had to endure my extreme tension.

The kids were usually good, but their perpetual arguments tore me apart. I found myself screaming silently at them, projecting on them the cold fury that I was feeling—which only made them worse. My daughter Mary, who began to perform poorly in school, was becoming morose and unmanageable. Sometimes when she looked at me, I felt that she hated me. That really grieved me because I wanted so badly for her to love me. Actually, I wanted everyone to love me, but I didn't think anyone did—except my husband, and I could never understand why. At one time we had seemed very close—or had that been just an illusion?

Every morning I awoke with that awful tight feeling that another day had to be endured. Would I make it? Would I be able to do all that was expected of me? The day would stretch far ahead of me, full of pitfalls which I would be very lucky to avoid. I feared that things would surely go wrong and I would feel very guilty.

Each night I found some escape from the ordeals of the day by reading, often until the early hours of the morning. Did I do that to devise some life that I could enjoy, even if it were not real, or was I denying myself the sleep that I felt I did not deserve? I cannot answer. Why did I dislike myself so much? I did not know the answer to that question either. I merely knew that I did not like my life as it was and desperately wanted it to change—although only a miracle could do that!

I heard that hypnosis was being used to relieve tension, and I knew that if I could just shed that awful tension, life would be easier. I was apprehensive and rather skeptical about the whole thing. Would it work for me? Would I be a failure at hypnosis as I was at so many other things? When I consulted my physician, he told me that hypnosis could help people learn to relax without the aid of drugs.

After some soul searching and with considerable trepidation, I eventually made an appointment to see Dr. Barnett. Very nervous as I was about that appointment, there were many times I found myself thinking of an excuse to break it. Was I so bad that I needed hypnosis? I was. I even recall sending my husband a card signed, "Your miserable wife!" But perhaps hypnosis was not for me. I had heard that not everyone could respond. In the end I did not break that appointment, and as events turned out I am very grateful to my guardian angel for making sure that I kept it.

During that first visit I was in a fog. I didn't notice much of the surroundings of the waiting room and was too tense to take heed of the gentle background music which I later realized was an integral part of the soothing atmosphere of Dr. Barnett's office. Only when I felt the warmth of the doctor's handshake did I begin to relax.

Glancing around his consulting room, I saw nothing unusual. I did not find any hypnotizing gadgets, but I was still too tense to notice very much. Later I recalled its well-lit, sunny appearance and the sounds of the traffic on the thoroughfare outside. I was sitting in an easy chair when Dr. Barnett returned to his desk.

When he asked what he could do for me, I began to feel that I had made a mistake and should not be there at all. I was looking for some excuse to leave as I murmured that I was afraid I was wasting his time. I did not feel that I could discuss all the things that were bothering me, so I just told him that my nerves were bad and that I was always tense.

Dr. Barnett seemed to understand that I really did not understand my irritability and unhappy moods. Before long I felt more at ease and was discussing my problems in a way which had previously been impossible.

Dr. Barnett pointed out how frequently I put myself down and asked if I knew why I did that. Somehow this had always seemed natural for me to do, but I told him I could not specify the motivation for it. He told me that I had learned to do this and that the impulse was probably concealed in my unconscious mind.

He went on to explain that hypnosis was simply a process of communicating with the inner mind whenever the conscious mind was sufficiently relaxed to allow that communication. Through the use of hypnosis he thought we might discover the reasons for my problems and solve them if I was prepared to cooperate. I must admit that I didn't feel cooperative at first, but as we talked, I began to experience a feeling of trust and eagerness to cooperate.

Continuing to speak in his soft, relaxing voice, Dr. Barnett asked me to close my eyes and completely relax my whole body. I felt myself drift into a very relaxed state, and I remember following his suggestion to imagine a very pleasant scene which seemed to be real and enjoyable. He continued to talk to me, and I know that I responded, but everything seemed vague and distant.

I heard him telling me to open my eyes and be wide awake. As I did so, I felt that I had awakened from a deep sleep and yet, paradoxically, it seemed as if I had simply closed my eyes for a few minutes. When I opened my eyes, I was aware that I had been crying, and yet I felt an enormous sense of relief—as if a tremendous burden had been lifted from my shoulders.

I experienced a mild sense of surprise when I looked at the clock and suddenly realized that I had been in his office for over an hour. Where had the time gone? What had been happening? I asked these questions of myself but was not concerned that I could find no immediate answer.

When Dr. Barnett asked how I was feeling, I told him that I was feeling great—and that surprised me. I wanted to laugh and sing—an extraordinary feeling. Dr. Barnett instructed me to return in one week. He told me that he believed that I would do very well, and somehow I felt sure that he was right.

As I made arrangements with his secretary for the next appointment, I could think of little but how good everything seemed. When I walked outside, the sounds and colors of the world seemed novel and interesting—as if I had never noticed them before. My senses were heightened in a wondering and wonderful way. I had always hated noises, but suddenly I was enjoying all of the bustle and clatter.

That was a memorable day for me. I can best describe it and the week that followed by quoting from my diary.

Tuesday

I sense that a mental and physical overhaul has begun since I saw Dr. Barnett. I feel literally wrung out, and yet I am serenely content. I felt so good this afternoon, that I found myself singing, "I'm sitting on top of the world."

All through the day this feeling of well-being has persisted. I have a strange sense that one part of me is quietly observing another.

Normally I'm a restless individual and can't sit quietly, yet this evening I'm resting quietly and comfortably, and the noise of the children's arguments is not angering me as it usually does. I feel relaxed and drowsy, without my usual desire to read and read.

Wednesday

I have enjoyed a day full of inner contentment—without the usual feelings of stress at all. I am aware of my usual angry or unhappy thoughts, but they are minimal and rapidly dissolve. I have the strange feeling that a new ME has arisen from deep inside and has taken control. It is like the angel of mercy has supplanted the devil. I am not frightened. In fact, I am at peace with myself for the first time in years.

Thursday

I am still happy and contented. I have had a marvelous time preparing and organizing Mary's birthday party. I was able to join in the fun of the party and had wonderful, warm feelings all the time. I am delighted at this new view. I like myself.

Friday

As I think of the changes that have occurred within me, I sense that I have at last become untangled and unwound. I suddenly feel as if I am no longer on trial, that everything that I am is acceptable. When I use those words "no longer on trial," I experience some strange feelings that I cannot identify.

Saturday

Patience, love and understanding have set the tone for today.

The children were home, and we have shared in so much fun and laughter. I am tapping new resources as the patience, love and understanding are far more pronounced. I have produced these attributes in the past, but not without great effort. Now I am not acting a role, for today these feelings flowed easily and spontaneously.

Sunday

I really blew it today! I believed that my personality was changing, but the "new being" was definitely not in charge. After experiencing several angry outbursts during the day, I am feeling very apprehensive.

Perhaps I can take some consolation from the fact that my anger was not as intense as it used to be, and it was never a cruel anger. Nevertheless, I feel really disappointed in myself, particularly since I cannot discover why I behaved this way. It seemed as if I just couldn't (or wouldn't) let that petulant mood go all day.

Monday

My thoughts aren't positive today. I feel that part of me is superimposing feelings upon another part of me and is striving for recognition. This would account for my actions yesterday. Today's discomforts have been triggered by the embarrassment of yesterday's outbursts, and I am trying to find answers to them. I must learn to accept my imperfections as well as my qualities; otherwise continuous discouragement is inevitable.

I will now leave my diary while I recall my next appointment with Dr. Barnett.

I was very uncertain whether I should relate how badly things seemed to go on Sunday, but in his office it seemed natural that I should discuss everything that happened. Dr. Barnett confirmed what I had already suspected—that the events on Sunday demonstrated that I have unpleasant as well as pleasant feelings, and that I am no better or worse than any other human being simply because I have these entirely normal human feelings.

I was particularly assured and relieved when Dr. Barnett pointed out that I had not used my anger aggressively or destructively, but only assertively. We talked about my positive feelings about myself and how I had actually begun to like myself. He then asked if I wished to reenter hypnosis. I agreed, and when he asked me to close my eyes, once again I felt that warm, peaceful and comfortable feeling drift over me as his relaxing voice continued.

Although I know that I listened to every word very carefully, it seemed only a few moments later that he was asking me to open my eyes and be wide awake. I sensed, even before I looked at the clock, that another hour had probably gone—and it had!

Dr. Barnett told me that he was very pleased at the progress I had made and that he was now confident that everything would be fine. In fact, he was so confident that he asked me to delay my next appointment for four weeks. I could not help feeling a little doubtful that I could remain well for four more weeks without help, but I tried not to show it.

Tuesday

Good feelings persisted today. I have felt confident, capable and self-assured. It seems as if I have relinquished many of my personal inhibitions. I am free—free to express feelings that I was previously compelled to hide.

For the first time in ages I was free to say the words "I love you" to my husband. Only I can appreciate the wonderment of being able to do that. The feeling has always been there, but the spoken words have given it such a profound meaning.

Wednesday

Today I feel the need for a deeper understanding of Mary. I want to earn her respect—not demand it. Becoming more aware of the interaction between us, I have tried to judge it objectively. My husband and I have discussed the problem this evening at length.

Through the remainder of my diary record of the four weeks between appointments I note that I have recorded some very interesting changes. I became more comfortable being myself. There seemed to be no further need to play any role or to do any pretending. It became O.K. to be me! I seemed to ease up and feel less pressure, yet I accomplished as much as before without any undue anxiety.

I began to look forward to each day. I stopped worrying about how I was going to cope. Unpleasant things continued to happen, but that seemed all right. I could deal with them in a controlled manner, accepting my uncomfortable feelings without experiencing guilt.

I became aware of a change taking place in my children and realized that they were responding to the modifications occurring in me. I was at last in harmony with the world.

There was still a doubting part of me which wondered whether this was all merely a dream from which I would shortly awaken. This doubt faded, however, with the passage of time, merely reminding me that I had never wanted the old me.

I began to delight in having unexpected guests drop by. Rather than panicking in my usual fashion, I enjoyed them—and I began to believe that they enjoyed me too!

One day my husband enthusiastically noted that he had been aware of a profound change in me since my first session of hypnotherapy. He had always wondered whether I had really loved him, but now the pronounced alteration in my outlook made it possible for him to broach the subject. He went on to confess that, over the years, he had found it difficult to speak to me about sensitive matters because I wouldn't express my hurt but always withdrew behind a wall of fury. I would walk around like a time bomb ready to explode, and thus no one dared approach me. I knew that he was right, for many times a disagreement between us aroused such intense feelings of hatred within me that I didn't dare to express them. And at such times I felt rejected by him.

I began to understand what had been boiling inside me during those years. I had been convinced that I was unlovable, that I couldn't give or receive love. I now know that this had never really been true. As a result, I can accept his love and give mine freely in return. The change has likewise had a profound effect upon Mary, who seems happier and more content.

Much happened in those four weeks between sessions. At times the old hate feelings returned and I felt afraid. But gradually I learned to talk my feelings out and became less afraid of them, particularly when I began to recognize that other people accepted my unpleasant feelings. After all, they shared them too!

When the four weeks were up, there was so much to tell Dr. Barnett that I hardly knew where to begin. After I confessed that I was still troubled by anger, he assured me that I would gradually come to accept it as a healthy part of me and no longer something to fear. I realize that he was right because each day I am finding my anger easier to accept and control.

He asked me to close my eyes and relax. Once again I drifted deeply into that interesting and pleasant state of awareness where internal thoughts and feelings assume such importance. This time it seemed as if I was there for a very long time. I recall his voice asking me if it would be all right for me to remember now, and my head nodded "yes."

When he asked me to open my eyes, my mind flooded with

131

painful memories. They were like scenes from a horror movie, but they were real—particularly a picture of a mother burning a little girl with a red hot poker. That mother was my mother, and the little girl was me. I could feel her terror. And then that horrible thing with dad. He should not have made me do that! I hate him and fear him— at least I used to. And then it was mother again—and always those men! Why couldn't I have a proper mother? I so wanted a proper mother!

I have now put all of those horrible pictures in their rightful place—into the past, where they no longer really matter. I have understood father. I understand mother. I no longer bear them any resentment, although I can never condone what they did to me. Most of all, I have forgiven myself. I now fully understand that all of us have a right to our feelings. It is not the feelings that are wrong, but the expression of feelings in a destructive manner.

I will always remember the three promises Dr. Barnett asked me to make to myself: never to put myself or my feelings down, never to allow anyone else to put me or my feelings down, and never to put anyone else or their feelings down. It all seemed marvelously clear and simple.

He asked if he could talk with my husband, so I brought him with me the following week. My husband admitted that some wonderful things had indeed happened, but he expressed a little of his own uncertainty as to whether such a tremendous change would be permanent. We all agreed that I should return for a follow-up appointment two months later.

I experienced a wonderful Christmas that year, and when I returned for my follow-up appointment in the new year, I reported that there had been no problems that I had not been able to handle. I had to admit that I was still a little uncomfortable when I thought about the past and the old me, but that visit was my last formal hypnotherapy. I had reached a stable understanding of myself and was fully able to accept myself as a worthwhile human being. I was really free!

Now, some three years later, I look upon these years as the happiest of my life. Each day seems as good as or better than the day before. Today the times of tension no longer seem overwhelming, and I am always confident that I can handle them.

I have devised a whole different set of values toward life. I feel relaxed with other people and no longer worry about what they will think of me. Interestingly enough, I have found that people seem to find it easy to accept me just as I am. Many of my friendships have become much deeper and more meaningful. I feel secure within myself and continue to enjoy self-confidence. I now have the ability to say "no" when asked to do something that I would prefer not to do, and I no longer experience any guilt feelings about my refusal.

To anyone seeking hypnotherapy I would say, "Do not be afraid." You may, as I did, discover unpleasant memories which you have spent your life filtering out of your mind without being able to escape feelings of guilt. You must allow yourself to face and deal with those memories, freeing yourself from their crippling effects on your life and happiness.

I am now able to look back at the old me without any distress because I realize that, without certain experiences, I would not be the person I am pleased to be today. I am surprised when people seek me out to help them with their problems, but Dr. Barnett tells me that this is because only an ex-convict can fully understand a prisoner. I know now what he means by that.

Dr. Barnett Comments:

Fortunately, H.B. was able to enter very deep hypnosis quickly. This enabled her to fully exploit her unconscious resources in the understanding of her problems. It also allowed her to deal rapidly with the critical experiences which had been responsible for the original crippling decisions she had made about herself. Early in life she had locked herself within the prison of anger. Deciding that she was a bad person and thus undeserving of love, she tried to smother any expression of anger or sadness. She even attempted not to feel these emotions. When she failed, an enormous sense of guilt overcame her.

In our very first session she was able to locate and recall the hurt and anger she had felt at her mistreatment. She could also understand that it really was not her fault. The discovery that she could accept her right to be herself, no matter what her feelings might be, instilled a positive attitude for the first few days after therapy. However, she had to try all of her feelings out, particularly when she had promised not to put them down or let anyone else deride them. At this time she became aware of insistent unpleasant feelings which clamored to be expressed. She learned that she could vent them without losing control of them.

Like many people who are able to enter a deep level of hypnosis, H.B. was able to forget the experiences which were recalled during the hypnotic state. Since she had this ability, I used it deliberately so that she was not initially forced to handle the memories in addition to the decisions that she had made. During the third session I asked her to remember all that had transpired in previous sessions—and she was able to deal with her past quite well.

The deep hypnosis which H.B. managed to reach enabled her to deal with her problems rapidly. In other examples of rapid resolution of problems, hypnosis has been much lighter. It usually takes longer to deal with problems when the level of hypnosis is not so deep, but as we shall see, the ultimate result is equally satisfactory.

2. M.E.

To her friends and family she was Mary, a well-meaning, practical woman who tried hard to be a perfect wife and mother. But deep inside Mary was a spontaneous, imaginative child named Elizabeth— that part of Mary which her mother could never tolerate.

Elizabeth longed to be loved and admired for herself, but Mary —without ever being aware of the tension fermenting within— repressed Elizabeth's wishes. Ever since she ceased to use the name Elizabeth as a child, Mary had known that her mother would only tolerate her if she gave up her deepest wishes and became compliant in all things.

As Mary grew older, early memories faded. By the time she wed, Elizabeth was nearly forgotten.

Mary's relationship with her husband was adequate as long as she deferred to his judgments at every turn. Occasionally she heard Elizabeth's rebellious voice crying out against this unequal regime, but Mary quickly silenced it. Another voice was needed to shatter the complacent life of the family.

Mary's mother-in-law accused Mary of dominating her husband because she didn't really care for him. Furthermore, she claimed that Mary had made herself a slave to her children. Such accusations left Mary in a state of shock. Having tried to nurture a spontaneous love for her husband, and deeply concerned for her children's welfare, she couldn't understand this attack.

In her home Mary's mother had dominated, badgering her husband and being unreasonably demanding of her children. Mary learned as a little girl to bury her anger toward her mother and to do everything possible to please her. She became artful at hiding her anxieties and presenting a personality that her mother could accept. Thrusting Elizabeth into the recesses of her consciousness when the pressures became too great, she adopted her second name, Mary, and attempted to conform.

Mary could not tell her mother-in-law how deeply the accusations had hurt and frightened her. One night, however, she awoke in an all-consuming rage toward the woman. Her fierce emotions confused and surprised her further, for she had always considered herself a gentle person. Now she was learning something about herself that did not fit the picture.

Mary had always been frightened of men. To be honest, she had never believed that any man would want her for his wife. Once married, she tried desperately to maintain her husband's (John) affection, fearing that he would leave her. She could not risk revealing Elizabeth's world to him.

Mary's emotional life with John seemed unfulfilling to her. His obstinacy and his inability to discover what was really important to her fixed a great gulf between them. Out of loneliness Mary developed a friendship with another man, who was able to sense the existence of Mary's inner world, the domain of Elizabeth. Torn by feelings of fear and exhilaration, Mary was relieved when the man moved away. Now she was safe from further discoveries which she feared she could not accept. But Elizabeth still longed for love and attention.

The long, hard winter wore down Mary's spirit. She feared that she would never survive the succession of icy grey days. The chill of the season seemed to squeeze the life from her, and she despaired of ever seeing another spring. Yet she clung to life. A voice inside whispered that she could not die—for she had never lived. In that desolate season she began to understand that she had done nothing for herself. She was always giving but never allowed herself to accept anything in return. Affection threatened her, fueling Elizabeth's determination to be acknowledged.

Spring brought Mary new hope and energy. She had survived. But the season also brought her new pain. A self-awareness class clarified for her the paradoxes she had recognized in her life. In the group she brought support and emotional nourishment to others but could accept none for herself.

Mary and John participated in a marriage encounter group during the summer. Throughout most of the sessions Mary wept. She felt as though she sat atop an emotional volcano due for eruption, but she couldn't locate the source of her pain. Slowly she became aware of needs that she could not fully understand. To express these emerging desires and feelings, she began to write poetry.

As a little girl Elizabeth had written poems and songs until her mother's dislike of her efforts had driven her creative needs inside. Now she returned to her poetry with a fierce, rebellious energy, and this brought her a feeling of wholeness she had not previously known.

But Mary could not allow anyone to read her writings. She could not share these new experiences with John, for she feared that his criticism would destroy the value of the poetry for her.

Mary attended another encounter group, and the pain that surfaced shattered her resolve to keep her anxieties hidden. Her poetry began to suffer. Fearful that this new source of wholeness in her life was about to be lost, she sought help with me.

I sensed early in our therapeutic relationship that Mary was desperate. She wanted to develop her independence from the obligations placed upon her by the family, but she equally sought to draw closer, emotionally, to her family.

Mary mentioned Elizabeth quite casually in our first session. She was surprised by my interest in her girlhood self and at first was confused when I asked whether Mary and Elizabeth were different people. She had never been able to appreciate the separateness of these two lives within her personality. Slowly Mary learned that it was Elizabeth who suffered pain, who needed to express herself in writing, who loved and hated fiercely and needed to be admired and cared for.

I suspected that some of Mary's problems could be traced right back to her birth experience. Therefore in our first session with hypnosis I asked her to regress to her natal hour.

"I feel sad," Mary told me when I asked her to explore her feelings at birth. "I feel as though I should never have come—never have been born. She doesn't want me. I see rubber gloves and a masked face, figures in white, then there is no one there. My mother is dead; I'm alone. I wish my father were here." At a later session she expanded her vision of that moment. "I thought I had killed her when I was born—she lay so cold and still under anesthesia. I felt impelled to give my life for her, to be whatever she wanted."

The experience of rejection and hurt was very strong for Mary. Sensing that her birth experience had left her with the feeling that she should not exist, I tried to impress upon her that she had a right to live—that it was OK to be.

When Mary freed herself from the feeling that she had killed her mother at birth, dramatic changes occurred in the way she related to her own body. She had associated her guilt and fear with the threatening violence of her breech birth. As she came to understand the natural conditions of her first few hours of life, her breathing became more relaxed. At the opening of our next session she exclaimed, "For many years I've undergone bouts of having to gasp for air. Suddenly I can breathe easily."

When Mary became more relaxed with her earliest memories, we progressed on to a time at which she was three years old. "I am little and I am in the water," Mary announced. "I am trying to decide whether to float out forever or to go back to shore. I decide to come back to land, but as I reach the shore, it is just as scary as the open water." She began to realize that even a child can harbor a death wish.

At ten Mary had an unfortunate, debilitating sexual experience with her father. "I see myself wearing my white saddle shoes," she reported. "I'm looking at my father's bare feet as he lies in bed. He wants me to come to him. Dad, I need you so much. Mother is killing me, but I am afraid of you."

I instructed Mary to use all her wisdom and inner strength to help that little girl. She responded slowly and fearfully.

In a later session Mary vividly recalled still another frightening sexual encounter with her father which required much encouragement to deal with.

In small, anxious steps Mary came to forgive the little girl Elizabeth. She learned that she needn't feel guilt for the molestation she suffered. In time she consciously recalled the assault by her father at five years of age, and her thoughts of that period began to emerge.

In one of our final sessions, Mary's feelings about her mother's fearful power over her became perfectly clear. She went quickly down to the level of hypnosis that most suited her and began to report what she saw and felt.

"It's my mother—her Royal Highness—again," she observed. "I think she must sit at the right hand of God. She is bending down to me and whispering, 'I don't love him, so you must.'"

I asked Mary what she would say to her mother.

"Love him yourself, you old witch," she replied with a thrill of anger. "That's your job, not mine."

As Mary worked through these problems over the next few months, many changes occurred in her life. She was able to write more freely and securely. Soon she could allow her poems to be read. She reported that her fear of men gradually diminished. She became much more self-assertive and enjoyed new sensations of emotional security. But nothing, she said, gave her more pleasure than the feelings of freedom she experienced.

One of Mary's anxieties concerned her son, Jason. He was a shy, retiring boy who was almost totally lacking in self-assurance. "It was as if he was afraid of his body. In hypnosis I was able to see the world through his eyes and discover that I was his problem. Because of my confusion about love and my own sexuality, I had rejected him since I had unconsciously felt it was wrong to love him in any physical way."

Mary was enormously relieved to learn that it was permissible to express all of her feelings toward her son. She began to hug and caress him as she had always wanted—with dramatic results. Jason blossomed out, becoming a more confident and open youngster.

Elizabeth had grown and matured during therapy until she was able to deal with life realistically rather than merely indulge her fantasies. Mary registered approval of Elizabeth's intuitive perceptions and relied increasingly upon the feelings of the inner personality.

Whenever a person changes his or her name, a subtle change in identity inevitably follows. This occurs when a woman marries and adopts her husband's family name or when a nickname is accepted or rejected. A name carries with it many unconscious associations, and thus the changing of one's name can result in the repression of some or all of its many associations. Thus when Elizabeth became Mary, she conformed to the behaviors expected of her and repressed the many feelings attributable to Elizabeth which were not acceptable to her mother.

Anyone who has a nickname can distinguish the different feelings generated by the nickname and the given name. Mothers must unconsciously recognize this fact when they use their children's full given name to address a serious problem rather than the pet name used for more frivolous matters.

Mary-Elizabeth's hypnoanalysis amply demonstrated the power of the sentence, "You must not exist," given for the crime of being born when unwanted. Her whole life prior to therapy had been dedicated to concealing part of herself from the world and exposing a front that was false but acceptable. This denial of her true self was inevitably the cause of much pain.

Mary's protection of Elizabeth was seen as necessary in order to avoid being abandoned. She did this by concealing Elizabeth and declaring to her that she had no rights whatever to herself or her feelings. Elizabeth's cries eventually became too strong to be suppressed when in the encounter group situation she realized that Mary was quite wrong. Every human being has a right to be loved.

Throughout therapy this right was stressed repeatedly. Whenever we located an experience which was rendering it difficult to retain acceptance of this fundamental right, we called upon her present increased knowledge and understanding to solve the difficulty. She was always successful.

Mary's history also emphasizes the importance of the birth experience in the development of an individual's concept of herself. In one of our later meetings, Mary relived her birth vividly. It was clear that she was experiencing a breech birth (i.e., a feet first birth) with all of the intense and frightening discomfort that a difficult breech birth must inflict upon a baby. There is always a period of suffocation, for instance, between the compression of the umbilical cord and the eventual emergence of the head which does not occur in a normal head first birth.

It was clear that much of Mary's fear of her mother began at this time, for her birth seemed like a life-and-death struggle between baby and mother, and she concluded that her mother had almost won. She could therefore never risk reengaging in battle with her mother. This accounted for the immense power that Mary's mother wielded over her through the years. To remain Elizabeth was to risk the annihilation that had almost occurred at birth.

Elizabeth's contemplation of suicide at the age of three probably arose from the unconscious feeling that mother's deeply needed approval could, in the last resort, be obtained by conceding victory and leaving the scene forever. Fortunately for Mary, she dealt with this problem by the excellent compromise of concealing Elizabeth and presenting her mother with the non-combatant Mary.

A very interesting feature of Mary-Elizabeth's story is the manner in which her children responded so dramatically to her therapy. It was quite apparent that the information regarding her children's problems and the solutions were available to her at an unconscious level. I have confirmed this on many occasions while treating other patients with problem children.

3. M.C.

Some people might have called me an alcoholic, but I would never have applied that label to myself. I would go for long periods without a drink but then, for no reason that I could discover, deliberately get very drunk and remain in that condition for a few days. As I look back on this period now, I recognize how I used to become increasingly depressed until I knew I was heading for another binge. Around the age of twenty-one I joined group drinking in bars. More recently I began to drink alone.

I have always been a loner, and yet a few dear friends really seem to care about me. Since I would do nothing to hurt them, I felt very ashamed when I knew how my drinking sprees affected them. I often promised my girlfriend that I would try to remain sober, but I always knew that I would let her down—and, of course, I did. At times, when I felt sure that I could lick my drinking problem, I could never understand why my resolutions proved to be so weak. I would have done anything to make her happy, but self-control seemed beyond me.

At her suggestion I called Dr. Barnett's office for an appointment to see if he could help, for he had been able to understand her smoking habit. During my first visit I underplayed my drinking problem because I had not been on a binge for two months and I was feeling that I really had it licked. Instead, I talked about another problem that I had experienced for years—feeling very uncomfortable with people, especially if more than two or three people were present. At parties I simply froze and couldn't wait to slip away unnoticed. I only went to parties because my friends thought I should.

Dr. Barnett asked me whether I felt that I did not belong. I agreed that this was exactly how I felt. On many occasions in a group I had sensed that I had nothing in common with any of them. It was almost as if they were talking a language I could not understand. Yet I know that I am a reasonably intelligent person and, although largely self-educated, possess a fair knowledge of the world around me. But I always felt inadequate when compared to everyone else, no matter who they were. I even felt inferior to my girlfriend at times, and she never did anything to put me down.

Dr. Barnett asked me if I liked myself. I had to consider that question carefully for a while. It was a new thought, but in the end I concluded that I really did not think highly of myself.

At the age of eighteen I was told by my parents that they had adopted me shortly after birth. They have always been very good to me, and I have always enjoyed a strong relationship with them. I do not think that the information about my adoption bothered me at all. Actually, I never thought much about my real parents.

When Dr. Barnett tested me for my ability to enter hypnosis, I feared that I would not be able to respond to any of his suggestions. Assuring me that I simply needed to relax, he asked me to close my eyes and let my unconscious mind give one signal for "yes" and another for "no." To my surprise, my right index finger lifted when I thought "yes," my right thumb when I thought "no." It was an uncanny feeling, particularly since I knew that I was wide awake. Dr. Barnett seemed to be satisfied, and he asked me to let my fingers move in any way they wanted.

He asked my unconscious memory to return to my birth, and I was surprised to feel my finger lift, indicating that my unconscious mind was there. I was shocked when it signaled that I had felt unwanted at my birth. Dr. Barnett went on to ask me if I felt guilty about being born, and my fingers answered with an emphatic "yes." Answers to further questions suggested that before I was born, I had heard my mother say that she did not want me at all. I was surprised and confused by these answers and wondered whether my unconscious mind could really be cooperating.

Dr. Barnett asked me if I could accept myself as a person as good and as important as any other human being. I remember that my "no" thumb lifted—and I was not surprised.

I was bewildered by my first visit, concluding that I had not been hypnotized at all. I could have opened my eyes at any time and walked out of the office—I am sure of that. But I found the involuntary movements of my fingers surprising. They seemed to have a life and mind of their own. To say that I was shocked by the answers they supplied would be an understatement.

I was eager to return for further therapy in order to hear what my unconscious mind would reveal through my fingers. At subsequent sessions I became convinced that my unconscious mind, with its amazing access to buried memories, was indeed answering Dr. Barnett's penetrating questions. We met every two weeks at first, later once a month. Dr. Barnett explained that the unconscious mind cannot be pushed. It will move at its own pace, and excessively frequent sessions accomplish no more than wisely spaced appointments.

In the first few meetings my unconscious mind consistently located all of my problems in the period before birth. It later went on to define my mother's rejection of me in even more positive terms. As time went on, I seemed to be hanging on to an intense hurt that resisted all of Dr. Barnett's effort to persuade me to relinquish.

Little by little I learned that my mother made three determined attempts to kill me before my birth. Unconsciously I was afraid of my mother and very angry with her. It seemed that I had dealt with this anger by focusing it upon myself. In other words, I was angry at myself for being born. I learned that by setting myself apart from the world, I was punishing myself for entering this world.

We later discovered an even deeper part of my unconscious self that was hurting very badly as a result of all this. This part desperately wanted to be a part of life but had discovered an escape from all of its pain through alcohol.

About this time in therapy I recognized the hopeless feeling that

I had always known just before going on an alcoholic binge, and it now made sense. I was using alcohol to "die" in the way I was supposed to have done before birth.

Three months after therapy began, we experienced the first real breakthrough. Dr. Barnett forced the punishing part of me to admit that I had been tormented long enough for allowing myself to live. However, he could not get it to agree to end punishment at that session.

At the very next session my unconscious mind indicated a clear image of my mother at my birth. She appeared to be dead, although she was probably only unconscious. It seemed as if I felt responsible for her "death" and had to go on punishing myself. Once again Dr. Barnett had great difficulty in persuading my unconscious mind that my mother was probably not dead and that, even if she were, I could not be held responsible.

More than six months after the commencement of therapy, my unconscious signals indicated a marked lessening of guilt and a real optimism about its eventual disappearance. During this period I drank only intermittently, and I noticed several other important changes occurring within me. I began to feel more relaxed in the company of others; during some periods I found myself feeling very good toward myself. At times I even asserted myself as I had never done before. I was beginning to be able to tell people exactly how I felt, whereas I had always kept my true feelings carefully hidden for fear that they would upset people. I now found that people were responding to me. It was an exciting, new feeling, and I was liking me.

More than nine months after we started therapy, the big day I had been waiting for arrived. My unconscious mind signaled that I had been completely forgiven and that there would be no further punishment. I was free at last. I could finally accept myself as a normal human being.

Since that day things have improved remarkably—so much so that I sometimes wonder if it has all been true. Of course, I still suffer "down" periods, but they are never bad enough to make me go on binges. I know that I will continue to drink occasionally, but I have an absolute conviction within me that I will never need to succumb to another binge. That, for me, spells freedom. I am enjoying each day that comes and no longer have any discomfort in a crowd of people. In fact, I rather like meeting new people, for I never seem to have difficulty finding something to talk about.

The last time that I visited Dr. Barnett's office I knew I wouldn't need to return. I had strong, positive feelings. Although I was certain then, as I am now, that problems would inevitably arise, I felt confident that I could deal with them without further help. I told Dr. Barnett that I had at last reached my objective and would not be returning unless I ran into a problem I could not handle.

Dr. Barnett Comments:

M.C.'s case illustrates that hypnoanalysis can help even the patient who is demonstrably an unsatisfactory hypnotic subject. Many hypnotherapists would have regarded M.C. as unhypnotizable because of his poor responses to suggestion. In spite of this, he was able to locate and deal with severe prenatal trauma—analysts would have considered this unthinkable a few years ago.

M.C.'s experiences had locked him up in the prison of guilt with the awful sentence "You must not exist" over his head. I know of no other therapy which could have successfully engineered his escape from this prison.

I learned from M.C. that no matter how black things appear initially during therapy, persistence will meet with success. He deserves commendation for persevering with therapy when the initial progress was slow. As one considers that the total period of therapy was less than a year, this does not seem to be so unusual, particularly when one hears of other less successful approaches to emotional problems taking several years to complete.

M.C. has remained well, and I believe that he will continue free from the need for alcoholic binges.

Chapter Fifteen

Healing

My whole life has been devoted to the study and the practice of healing. Unfortunately, however, a physician spends a great deal of his time studying disease and insufficient time investigating health. The diseases are so numerous and complex that they occupy most of his thinking. He comes to regard disease as an enemy which must be hunted down and destroyed. In the case of the infective diseases, of course, this is a very rational approach, following naturally upon the older concept of devils inhabiting the body and causing disease.

Infective organisms can often be detected by modern techniques, and in these days of antibiotics many specific agents are available for their destruction. This approach has proved to be so enormously successful in many of the infective diseases that modern medicine tends to ignore the defenses which the body has evolved over the centuries of man's development to combat such infections. It is true that these defenses may be overwhelmed by the severity of the infection, and the intervention of specific therapy has wrought miracles in thousands upon thousands of cases in recent years. I deplore the tendency of modern medicine to ignore the role of the body's defenses in dealing with disease. This is particularly important when we look at the non-infective diseases, since our control of these remains disappointing.

The progress of modern obstetrics has been marked by a tendency to ignore the body's own inherent defenses and to replace them with man-made appliances and intervention so that the body's ability to handle normal childbirth is hampered by drugs, surgical intervention and negative suggestions. Such interventions, we are told, make childbirth safer for the mother and the child, but under closer scrutiny this rationale has recently been found to carry much less truth than would at first appear.

As a general physician with a long experience of successful home deliveries where interference in the normal processes of childbirth were minimal, I applaud the efforts of those who oppose the increasing mechanization of obstetrics. I do so on the basis of the belief implicit throughout this book—that we possess resources to deal with our problems so long as we allow ourselves to call upon them.

145

Our symtomatic control of disease is improving steadily so that by the use of drugs and surgery we can secure a measure of comfort where before there was none. But the non-infective diseases, which include cancer, heart disease, psychosomatic diseases and the degenerative disorders, continue to pose problems in therapy which have yet to be resolved.

Medical science understands some of the mechanisms by which the body conducts its healing. The action of the leucocytes in devouring foreign invaders is certainly well-documented, and the formation of specific enzymes to promote chemical changes favorable for healing and the production of antibodies to help immobilize the antagonists have also been subjected to intensive study. Not clearly understood is the wide variation of healing responses in different individuals so that in an epidemic of an infective disease, some will survive unscathed and others will succumb. Also, we do not know why non-infective diseases will occur more readily in some individuals than in others.

Without a doubt, the psychosomatic disorders reflect a distinct emotional background. It is also agreed that personality plays a part in cardiovascular diseases and even in such a purely physical phenomenon as proneness to injury. There is even some evidence to support the contention that cancer sufferers have a tendency towards a guilt ridden, negative personality.

This suggests that disease is very much influenced by mental attitudes. Every physician at some time in his career has met the patient whose recovery from an illness has been unduly prolonged. In such people a "will to die" retards recovery and may even effectively prevent it. Physicians have frequently been amazed at the rapidity with which some determined individuals will recover from a severe illness or surgical procedure.

These findings indicate that the unconscious mind can play a direct part in the process of healing. Our unconscious resources are still only vaguely understood and remain largely untapped. Those of us who work with hypnosis have accrued experience with patients who, under the influence of hypnotic suggestion, have made an unusual recovery from chronic illnesses which have defied conventional therapy.

It has also been conclusively proven that the body will heal much more rapidly from minor injuries and burns if hypnotic suggestion is used as an element of the therapy. The unconscious mind is presumably paying closer attention in hypnosis to what is being said than it would normally.

Patients who have been given instructions to heal while under an anesthetic will often do better than those who have not been given such suggestions. Dentists who administer suggestions in hypnosis have repeatedly noted the decrease in bleeding and discomfort that occurs after dental surgery. They have also observed that the gums heal very quickly.

Suggestion's potent effect on recovery is labeled by orthodox medicine as the placebo effect. Whenever any medication or procedure is administered with the expectation that it will have a given effect, a proportion of patients will indeed experience that effect regardless of the medication employed. In some cases it appears sufficient only for the patient to believe that the medicine will produce the desired effect for it to occur. This "placebo" effect makes it extremely difficult to evaluate the intrinsic value of a new drug in human beings. Totally inert sugar pills, for instance, have been effective in relieving severe post-operative pain in about thirty percent of patients who believed that they were receiving strong pain-relieving medication.

How the unconscious mind can carry out these instructions to promote healing is still somewhat of a mystery, although some evidence suggests that it operates via the autonomic nervous system—that part of the nervous system which, though very complex, is not under conscious control. All examples of faith healing may act in this manner, for there is always the hope, as well as the expectation, of healing prior to the ceremony, which provides the signal for the unconscious mind to set the healing process in motion.

It has long been known that warts can be cured by various procedures recorded in folklore. Once again it is probable that the expectation of healing initiates the unconscious mechanisms. In the case of warts we can speculate that, by controlling the blood vessels to the warts and reducing the supply of blood in the area, the unconscious mind causes them to die from starvation. We know that this particular mechanism is possible since blanching of the skin due to constriction of the blood vessels in the skin following appropriate suggestions is demonstrable in certain people.

More recently we have learned that some people dying of "incurable" cancer have been able to arrest and even reverse the progress of their disease by using imagery techniques similar to those utilized in self-hypnosis.

In all cases where suggestion, however applied, effects healing, we can assume that the resources for healing were already present but were either not being used at all or were insufficiently mobilized. The suggestion then merely encourages the body to fully activate its available resources.

Hemophilia, a well-known bleeding disorder, results from an hereditary deficiency of an important clotting factor. This factor may be more deficient at some times than others, which accounts for the periodicity of the disease. Suggestion in hypnosis will encourage the body to increase the amount of the deficient factor sufficiently to control bleeding. Hemophiliacs therefore can use this mechanism in addition to unconscious control of damaged blood vessels to regulate bleeding when subjected to injury.

In light of all the evidence available to twentieth century science we must ask, Why do we not always fully use our unconscious resources for healing? Quite possibly the body's normal healing resources are unconsciously inhibited in certain cases. But when analytical methods are applied, a need for self-punishment, resulting from unresolved feelings of guilt, may be uncovered. Such a need will account for the "will to die" that I have already mentioned.

Only by the resolution of emotional problems which may still exist at the unconscious level can the inhibition of the unconscious resources for healing be removed and normal healing established. Fortunately, communication with the unconscious mind is facilitated by hypnosis, and suggestions given in this unconsciously attentive state can, when acceptable, be extremely effective.

Since we must recognize that drugs and surgery will never provide the answer to more than a significant minority of disorders, it is hoped that orthodox medicine will eventually recognize that the enormous potential of the unconscious mind for healing is available for the asking. It is my sincere hope that all of the avenues for tapping these resources will eventually be fully researched. An even more effective means of accomplishing this than by the use of hypnosis may eventually be discovered.

Chapter Sixteen

Summing Up

Freedom is the birthright of every human being, but many of us have never felt freedom and do not realize that we have a right to it.

In these pages I have tried to charter the pathway that I have found to freedom, one which I hope many will be encouraged to follow.

On my consulting room wall hangs a copy of Frederick Perls' Gestalt prayer. I turn to it whenever I encounter any difficulty in conducting my patients out of their mental prisons to freedom:

I do my thing and you do your thing
I am not in this world to live up to your expectations
And you are not in this world to live up to mine
You are you and I am I
And if by chance we find each other
It is beautiful

These words sum up what I try to do in hypnotherapy and indicate the route that I take with my patients.

I do my thing and you do your thing.

Few of my patients can fully understand this first phrase. All too frequently they are not aware of an "I." They have so repressed the Child within themselves that this phrase makes no sense to them. And without an "I," one can have no "thing."

Much of our initial work together is taken up with discovering the "I" and determining his "thing." Here the initial uncovering techniques of analytical hypnotherapy are extremely important. By determining the critical experiences when the "I" was hidden, we can make the change from imprisonment to freedom.

I am not in this world to live up to your expectations. Most of my patients have geared their lives to the expectations of others—especially mother. This thought comes as a blinding revelation to them, for they have never before considered that there could be any other reason for existence. Yet it is only when one ceases to live up to the expectations of others that the gates to freedom begin to swing open and the chains of guilt fall away. This idea is so new to people that only the next sentence enables them to accept it—*And you are not in this world to live up to mine.* The fairness of this phrase is strikingly irresistible.

In this phrase appears the essential equality of man which is also stressed by the next phrase. *You are you and I am I.* Such an affirmation expresses the essential importance and goodness of human beings which is stressed during therapy. In it can be heard the sense of purpose in each human being's existence which is underlined by the final phrase, *And if by chance we find each other it is beautiful.* Life is just a series of chances, yet its purpose is defined by the chance meeting of independent, free, important, self-accepting individuals. The beauty of these meetings cannot be described. It can only be felt. Freed prisoners can experience this beauty and the happiness it brings many times each day.

Although this book demonstrates the way in which analytical hypnotherapy can be used to gain freedom, hypnosis is only one of the many ways in which an escape from the prisons of the mind can be effected. Many religions can attest to the fact that self-acceptance has led to the beauty of freedom. My main goal has been to show that many of us are living needlessly impoverished lives. We are wasting time which could be lived fully.

Critics of the analytical approach to therapy have repeatedly insisted that the past is finished, that we should forget it and get on with living in the present. I have no quarrel with this point of view. However, analytical hypnotherapy recognizes that many of us are unconsciously bound to and ruled by our past, which prevents us from living fully in the present. The free individual is unshackled from his past. His former days serve as interesting history, nothing more. They no longer have the power to prevent him from responding to the present simply and honestly. He has no further need to protect himself from the past.

The freed individual can fully respect all of his internal responses. They are good, God-given—present in all of us to protect and guide us, each keeping us informed about the world in which we live. Although we represent varying viewpoints, we can agree to respect both our views and those of our fellow human beings.

Freed individuals become much more tolerant of their fellows. They always appear to be at peace with themselves and do not make undue demands upon others. They are able to accept pain and deal with it. As highly self-protective people, they never allow anyone to cause them to devalue themselves. Not believing in essential evil, they are aware that prisoners in torment will endeavor to inflict some of their pain upon their fellows. They firmly believe that the world would indeed be at peace should each human being fully accept himself.

My work with analytical hypnotherapy has taught me the

tremendous importance of the mother/child relationship. It has repeatedly emphasized that problems occur when a child has felt rejected by its mother following conception and indicates that a race of free people will probably never really arise until we can create a race of free mothers—mothers who really accept and respect themselves as people.

Some Thoughts on Loneliness

Everyone is alone. Few of us are "all one." But when we become all one, we no longer feel lonely, even when we are alone.

Loneliness results from rejection of part of the self so that one portion feels cut off, isolated and afraid. To banish loneliness, we need to be totally and unreservedly self-accepting. We can then become and remain all one. This will be difficult if, when rejected by others, we reject ourselves.

We therefore need to continue to accept ourselves in the face of rejection by others. We must not depend upon their acceptance in order to gain self-approval.

When we become aware of our motivation for craving acceptance by others, often at the cost of self-rejection, we discover the means to free ourselves from that need. The exorbitant price of self-rejection, that of emotional and physical ill health, need no longer be paid.

Some Thoughts on Responsibility

Within our personalities certain assets and liabilities form an integral part of nature. We alone are responsible for the person we are, and we cannot transfer that responsibility to anyone else. We are also accountable for our actions and feelings; we cannot blame them on others.

The freed individual accepts his fundamental responsibilities, whereas the prisoner of the mind constantly seeks to assign his to others. The freed individual refuses to accept the responsibilities of another since he believes in the ability of each individual to fulfill his own responsibilities.

Although a freed individual may respond to another person's actions with feelings of anger, hurt or fear, he does not blame that person for his discomfort. He accepts responsibility for it himself and deals with it appropriately. Conversely, should his own actions result in a negative response from another person, he may rue that fact, but he will not accept responsibility for it and is under no pressure to resolve it.

The freed individual can be of great help to his comrades since he never seeks to find solutions to their problems but instead encourages them to use their own resources to resolve personal problems.

Some Thoughts on Loving

To love someone is to be at peace with them. The greater the peace, the greater the love. Loving cannot exist in the presence of anger, for anger inevitably disrupts peace. However, it is always possible to dissolve anger and to return to loving.

Frequently confused with needing, which creates a demanding relationship in which peace is a rare ingredient, loving makes no demands upon anyone. It is totally accepting of the person loved.

The freed individual first and foremost is at peace with himself and therefore loves himself. He is totally self-accepting. Because of this, he does not constantly need to be comforted. This demand for comforting is often confused with love by those who are imprisoned.

Because he is at peace with himself, the freed individual will enjoy a tranquil relationship with many of his fellow human beings. He is able to love them, and his capacity for loving is limitless.

Living is loving. The person who cannot love is dead. The freed individual is living because he never ceases loving.

Some Thoughts on Equality in Human Beings

The philosophy upon which analytical hypnotherapy is based stresses the basic goodness and uniform importance of humanity. The complexity of human beings makes them the most wonderful product that we know of in this truly wonderful universe. The differences among us all, which reflect the extreme complexity of each human being, are minimal—and relatively insignificant. The tendency to regard the wealthy, the clever, the beautiful or the strong as "more equal" than others must be resisted, for it clouds the recognition of the basic fact of human similarity and importance.

Each of us enters and leaves this world in the same way. The style of our entrance and exit will differ, but this variance is not under our control. We all possess similar mental, physical and emotional equipment which differs in detail only. The philosophy of basic human equality is fundamental to successful therapy.

The freed individual's acceptance of his equality with his fellow human beings liberates him from the compulsion to prove himself better than others. Thus he is a totally integrated personality, deriving energy from the Child, nurturing from the Parent and control from the Adult.

BIBLIOGRAPHY

Alberti, R.E. & M.L. Emmons. *Your Perfect Right.* San Luis Obispo, California: Impact, 1970.

Arms, Suzanne. *Immaculate Deception.* Houghton Mifflin, 1975.

Berne, Eric. *Transactional Analysis in Psychotherapy.* Grove Press Inc., 1961.

Berne, Eric. *What do you say after you say hello?.* Grove Press Inc., 1972.

Berheim, H. *Hypnosis and Suggestion in Psychotherapy.* Jason Aronson Inc., 1973.

Birnbaum, Jack. *Cry Anger.* General Publishing Co., Ltd., 1973.

Branden, Nathaniel. *The Disowned Self.* Nash Publishing Corporation, 1972.

Cheek, David & LeCron Lesie. *Clinical Hypnotherapy.* Grune & Stratton.

Flach, Frederic R. *The Secret Strength of Depression.* J.B. Lippincott, 1974.

Harris, Thomas A. *I'm O.K. You're O.K.* Harper & Row, 1967.

Hull, Clark L. *Hypnosis and Suggestibility.* D. Appleton-Century Company Inc., 1975.

Hilgard, Ernest R. *The Experience of Hypnosis.* Harcourt Brace & World Inc., 1968.

Hilgard, Ernest R. *Divided Consciousness.* John Wiley & Sons, 1977.

Leonidas, Professor. *Secrets of Stage Hypnotism.* Newcastle Publishing Company Inc., 1975.

Marks, I.M. *Fears and Phobias.* Heinmann London, 1969.

Perls, Fritz. *The Gestalt Approach.* Science & Behaviour Books, 1973.

Peterfy, George, *Hypnosis,* Chapter 13, "Psychosomatic Medicine." Harper & Row, Edited by Wittkower & Warnes. Harper & Row, 1967.

Rubin, Theodore I. *Compassion and Self Hate.* David McKay Co., Inc. New York, 1975.

Seabury, David. *The Art of Selfishness.* Julian Messner, 1964.

Simonton, O.C., Matthews-Simonton S. & Creighton J. *Getting Well Again.* J.P. Tarcher. Los Angeles, 1978.

Stein, E.V. *Guilt: Theory and Therapy.* George Allen & Unwin Ltd., London, 1969.

Tec, Leon. *The Fear of Success.* Reader's Digest Press, 1976.

ANALYTICAL HYPNOTHERAPY
Principles and Practice
Edgar A. Barnett, M.D.

Analytical Hypnotherapy is a unique blend of analytic and direct suggestion techniques, grounded in a perspective that makes perfect sense. Each practitioner can integrate various aspects of the system into his or her existing therapy techniques, utilizing them to maximize and improve results without making radical changes to an established approach.

Clearly written and well researched, the book is detailed in its explanation of theory and very effective in its explanation of practice.

The first section reviews such subjects as the history of hypnoanalysis, the nature of hypnosis, and a range of techniques especially for rapid induction in both children and adults. The second section deals primarily with case histories and forms a major part of the work. A wide range of topics is covered, including negative birth experience, sexual dysfunction, obesity, migraine, smoking, alcoholism, and phobias.

"Rich clinical vignettes provide opportunity for the reader to experience the way this technique is applied."

American Journal of Clinical Hypnosis

- Hard cover • More than 500 pages • $37.50
- Illustrations and tables • Preface by David B. Cheek, M.D.
- Annotated case histories • Extensive bibliography
- Subject index • Name index

Ask about our FREE VIDEO
"Hypnotherapy as a Career"

"Hypnotherapy as a Career" Training in Clinical Hypnosis and Hypnotherapy

- Accelerated Intensives (50 hours in five days) or Weekend Classes (10 hours each Saturday)

- Diplomas awarded as "Master Hypnotist," "Hypnotherapist" and "Clinical Hypnotherapist"

- All diplomas authorized by the California Board of Education

- Approved by the California Board of Behavioral Science Examiners and the California Board of Registered Nursing

- National certification awarded

- One-, two-, three-, and four-week programs available

For details on this exciting and rewarding profession
write for our **free** catalog:

Hypnotism Training Institute of Los Angeles
700 S. Central Ave., Dept. TT
Glendale, CA 91204
or call
(818) 242-1159

HYPNOTISM TRAINING VIDEOS

NEW INSTANTANEOUS INDUCTIONS

TWO SUBJECTS; Total Loss of Equilibrium; Eye Catalepsy/Arm Catalepsy; Deepening by Compounding; Deepening by Reinduction; Non-Verbal Reinduction; The Myth of "Special Inductions"; Waking Hypnosis Creating Partial Amnesia; Creating Total Post-Hypnotic Amnesia; Normalizing Suggestions; Induced Speech Inhibition; Second Instantaneous Induction; Test Eye Catalepsy; Rule of Reversed Mental Effort; Teaching Self-Hypnosis to Subject; Healing Suggestions; Trance Termination.

FREE BONUS

COLIN - A student from England has never been hypnotized before. Gil Boyne demonstrates Instantaneous Induction (standing), deepening by disorientation, eye catalepsy, deepening by realization, rule of reverse mental effort, deepening by rocking subject, arm catalepsy, deepening by compounding, automatic motion, deepening by pyramiding, had-clasp response, creating somnambulism, creating post-hypnotic proof-of-trance, conditioning for post-hypnotic reinduction by repeated instant inductions, post-hypnotic talk, post-hypnotic reinduction, why *"fully aware"* replaces *"wide awake"*, trance termination, second post hypnotic talk.
Instantaneous Inductions and Colin (FREE BONUS)
49 minutes • $49.95

NEW MOLLY: SEATED INDUCTIONS

A variety of seated induction techniques with one subject. Includes conscious and subconscious re-education. Numerous deepening and conditioning techniques.
58 minutes • $49.95

HYPNOTISM TRAINING FILM #501
GIL BOYNE TEACHING AND DEMONSTRATING

Hypnotherapist, Gil Boyne demonstrates five methods of Instantaneous Induction and simultaneously explains the processes in non-technical language as he works with ten subjects.

Vivid examples of *Testing and Deepening, Training the Client, Developing Rapid Rapport and Reeducating the Client* are captured live and unrehearsed, using students in attendance. Also includes Arm Levitation, Eye Catalepsy, Arm Catalepsy, Automatic Motion, Key Word Reinduction. Plus ten methods of deepening the trance, post-hypnotic suggestions, and amnesia and other hypnotic phenomena.
105 minutes Special Offer - Our best selling video at a special price: Was $125.00 - now just $39.95. Includes a complete word-for-word transcript of the film absolutely FREE!

GIL BOYNE'S
HYPNOTISM TRAINING FILM #300
Part I Advanced Hypnotic Training

Actual live, unrehearsed demonstrations filmed in a classroom setting using the students in attendance. Gil Boyne teaches and demonstrates Instantaneous Inductions, Testing and Deepening, Training the Client, Developing Rapid Rapport, Reeducation of the Client.
Part II How To Visualize

A frustrating problem for hypnotherapists is the number of clients who report they are unable to visualize or use visual imagery. Here is how you can finally overcome that problem -- forever.

At a training seminar a student informs Gil Boyne that he is unable to visualize. Watch as Boyne hypnotizes the subject and creates a process in which the subject "sees, hears, tastes, feels and smells."
105 minutes • $65.00

STAGE HYPNOSIS

PART ONE - From 1960 to 1965, Gil Boyne entertained thousands with his *"Hilarious Hypnosis Stage Show"* in nightclubs throughout the U.S.A. This video tape combines one full hour of highly-skilled stage hypnosis techniques with the hilarious antics of a stage full of subjects.

PART TWO - Ormond McGill, Dean of American Hypnotists, presents a fascinating and mirth provoking one-hour show in his unique style. This is your opportunity to compare and learn from the art of two of the world's great stage hypnotists.
120 minutes • $79.95

WEIGHT LOSS

THE PSYCHOLOGY OF WEIGHT LOSS

Here is a videotape that helps you slim down from the inside. Starting with the confessions of overweight people (all but one of whom are women) about their eating disorder, we move to advice from clinical hypnotherapist John Zulli and counselor Pamela Scott. Using close-ups almost exclusively, the tape offers personal revelations about emotional eating, subconscious programming, body image, and low self-esteem, as well as childhood abuse traumas. The candid self-analyses and subsequent interpretations by Zulli and Scott are informative and inspirational. The tape offers good advice - it acts as sort of an individual therapy session. Technical qualities are professional, especially the client editing work.
47 minutes • $29.95
(Review -- Library Journal 04-15-93)

MARKETING YOUR HYPNOTISM SERVICES

GIL BOYNE'S
"HOW TO TEACH SELF-HYPNOSIS"
Hypnotherapists—
Here's How to Double Your Income!
The Complete Course on Video Cassette

Since 1956, Gil Boyne has taught self-hypnosis to more than 23,000 persons in Southern California. Boyne drew from his vast background of experience to create his most exciting new project - - a comprehensive course on "How To Teach Self-Hypnosis" -- eight hours of actual teaching on video cassette.

See and hear every element in the successful teaching of self-hypnosis, skillfully demonstrated in an actual class setting.

The videos also include a 99-page Marketing Manual and a complete word-for-word transcript of the eight-hour video cassette.

8 hours • 4 video tapes PLUS two manuals • $195.00
Also available separately: "How To Teach Self-Hypnosis" Transcript/Training Manual, $35.00; and Marketing Manual, $35.00; Both manuals for $50.00

HYPNOSIS FOR HEALING AND PAIN CONTROL

HYPNOSIS FOR MEDICAL EMERGENCIES

Using spontaneous hypnosis to communicate with the sick and injured to control pain and enhance recovery. Why is it that conversation at the scene of a medical emergency can have such a critical effect on the patient? This video shows that it is because frightened or seriously injured persons spontaneously enter into a hypnotic state of consciousness that makes them acutely responsive to certain kinds of direct or indirect suggestions.

This program uses dramatizations and graphic illustrations to present guidelines, strategies and techniques for gaining rapport and for giving suggestions and directives that can remarkably help patients control their own autonomic nervous system responses. These include:

- Bleeding
- Blood Pressure
- Respiratory Functions
- Burn Injury Reaction
- Pain Response
- Immune Response
- Inflammation
- Heart Rate
- Dermatitis

50 minutes • $69.95

"Don Jacobs video presents proof positive that the use of appropriate words in critical situations can not only speed healing but save lives as well.
Gil Boyne
Exec. Director, American Council of Hypnotist Examiners

"Dr. Jacobs' approach to pre-hospital care has the potential of having a great impact on treatment outcomes."
Alan V. Brunacini
Chief, Phoenix Fire Dept.

"As this use of hypnosis is extended there will be many lives saved."
David Cheek, M.D.
Author, Clinical Hypnotherapist

"This tape is on the cutting edge of an exciting and innovative approach to pre-hospital care."
Bennie Cooper, M.A.
R.E.M.T.
Director of Emergency Medical Training, Murray State University

FREE BONUS
HOW TO USE HYPNOSIS IN A HOSPITAL SETTING

Gil Boyne and respiratory therapist Jack Silvas demonstrate the use of trance for pain control and overcoming patients' poor sleep patterns, plus how to teach the use of hypnotic cassettes by the patient for pain control. (95 photographic slides with narration on video tape)

42 minutes • FREE BONUS with the purchase of Hypnosis For Medical Emergencies.

CLINICAL HYPNOTHERAPY

HOLLY ("YOU SCARE ME") and
PAT ("FEAR OF PUBLIC SPEAKING")

Holly, a young woman in her mid-twenties, breaks into tears in the first day of a Clinical Hypnotherapy course. When instructor Gil Boyne questions her she says, "You're scaring me." This seems a paradox since Boyne has not spoken directly to her in the class. He suggests that he hypnotize her to discover the background of her emotional upheaval. In minutes she is regressed to a terrifying scene with a threatening step-father. Abreaction, reeducation, rescripting and closure occur in rapid succession and the projected fear of an animated authority figure is dissipated.

PART TWO - A mature, intelligent female hypnotherapy student reports a fear of public speaking. She states that she "always sounds haughty" when speaking to a group. A comprehensive intake interview fails to reveal any evidence of negative childhood experiences or identifications. Trance is induced and deepened and a highly specialized program of affirmations and visualizations is presented.
75 minutes • $45.00

NEW THE CASE OF "BUNNY"
PHYSICAL PAIN FROM EARLY SEXUAL ABUSE

Boyne demonstrates instantaneous inductions with several subjects. While testing one of them by making her upraised arm rigid she exclaims, "It's a miracle." She goes on to say that she has been unable to lift her arm higher than her shoulder for over two years. Boyne hypnotizes her and in an exciting and highly dramatic age-regression he discovers the cause of her arm, neck, and shoulder problems to be a result of early sexual abuse by her alcoholic father. Using several original and unorthodox techniques, Boyne creates a complete release from these disabling symptoms.
58 minutes • $95.00

NEW THE FEAR OF CRITICISM & THE CURSE OF PERFECTIONISM

Gil Boyne lecturing teaches the crippling effects of the fear of criticism and the style of perfectionism. He works with two subjects (Miriam, Sam); and discovers "childhood scripts" including the compulsive people-pleaser, "Won't Say No."
53 minutes • $49.95

NEW GEORGE/BOB

OVERCOMING THE *"I CAN'T BE HYPNOTIZED"* PROBLEM. George, a university professor from Connecticut, has been many years in the practice of hypnosis but still doesn't know if he has ever been "in a trance" or if his clients have ever been hypnotized. One session with Boyne convinces him of his trance-state to his satisfaction.

"FEAR OF FAILURE" Bob, a 72 year old Hypnotherapist has been unable to experience trance despite his many efforts to do so. Using age regression, Boyne uncovers mother's early scripts "You'll never amount to anything". Bob enters into a deep trance complete with several tests. Boyne then teaches him self-hypnosis and he comes up from the trance amazed and radiant.
100 minutes • $95.00

THE CASE OF BUD
("BORN TO LOSE")

A depressed male in his mid-fifties is convinced that he is a loser in life. Suffers from alcoholism, insomnia, low self-esteem, self-isolation and negative thinking. In two one-hour sessions on consecutive days, Bud experiences an amazing personal transformation. Filmed live before a hypnotherapy class of forty-five therapists in Chicago. Shows age-regression, abreaction, Gestalt dialogues and many of Gil Boyne's original uncovering/reprogramming techniques.
95 minutes • $75.00

THE CASE OF LEE
("THE SAN DIEGO STUTTERER")

In a dramatic two hour hypnotherapy session using age regression and "uncovering techniques" Gil Boyne unveils the "battered child" syndrome and fear of castration as an initial sensitizing event for a life-long pattern of stuttering. Three years later, Lee remains totally free of stuttering. Gestalt dialogues, bodywork techniques and Parts therapy.
120 minutes • $75.00

BEST SELLERS

SUCCESS THROUGH MIND POWER
How to Be a Winner in the game of Life
Roy Hunter, M.H.

Why is change so elusive? Because we are often told what to change but never taught how. Now there is a step-by-step course in how to make the changes you desire through Mind Power Exercise, a simple and systematic approach to positive action that can help ensure success in every aspect of life.
Paperback • $6.95 • 130 pages

FINANCIAL SUCCESS THROUGH CREATIVE MIND POWER
(The Science of Getting Rich)
Wallace D. Wattles

This small book is a practical manual intended for men and women whose most pressing need is for money; who wish to get rich first and philosophize after. It has been responsible for the success of thousands of Mind Power students in the half-century since it was first published.
Paperback • $6.95 • 92 pages

HYPNOTISM AND MYSTICISM OF INDIA
Ormond McGill

Noted author and hypnotist McGill reveals how the real mysticism and magic of India are accomplished. His detailed instructions for developing the powers of Oriental hypnotism are drawn from the secret teachings of the Masters of India, where he lived and studied for several years.
Hardcover, Illustrated • $18.95 • 203 pages

UNLOCK YOUR MIND AND BE FREE WITH HYPNOTHERAPY
Edgar A. Barnett, M.D.

Written by a medical doctor who now practices exclusively as a hypnotherapist, this dramatic book presents fascinating case studies in which hypnosis is the demonstrated key to solving emotional difficulties. Includes sections on self-hypnosis and self-analysis, and age regressions.
Paperback • $8.95 • 155 pages

TOTAL MIND POWER
Donald L. Wilson, M.D., Certified Hypnotherapist

How you can unlock the secrets to better health and happiness. Dr. Wilson's best-selling book teaches you easily learned, powerful techniques for tapping the other 90% of your mind.
Hardcover • Illustrated • 254 pages • $9.95

THE MIRACLE OF MIND POWER
Dan Custer

Enjoy better health, greater happiness and increased prosperity through the dynamic power of your mind. This stimulating and inspiring book is full of methods for tapping that power which you can start putting to work immediately.
Paperback • 263 pages • $7.95

HYPNOTHERAPY
Dave Elman

In this major work Elman creates a forceful and dynamic presentation of hypnosis as a lightning-fast and amazingly effective tool in a wide range of therapies. A summary of Elman's theories and techniques, it is a classic in the literature on hypnotism.
Hardcover • 336 pages • $27.50

HYPNOTISIM & MEDITATION
Ormond McGill, Certified Hypnotherapist

An operational manual for Hypnomeditation. Every process is clearly explained and detailed formulas are given. Fifteen days with Hypnomeditation will change your life!
Paperback • 99 pages • $6.95

THE NO -SMOKING BOOK
How To Quit Through Self-Hypnosis
Isabel Gilbert

Endorsed by many prominent doctors, Gilbert's simple method uses self-awareness, self-hypnosis, relaxation and self-programming, each taught in a clear, precise and good-humored style. Practical

suggestions deal with the temptations of backsliding.
Paperback • $6.95 • 84 pages

SELECTIVE AWARENESS
Peter Mutke, M.D.

A step-by-step series of easily understood procedures for making contact with and between our various physical and mental parts and functions so we may gain more control over our own health. Includes pain control, accelerated healing, weight reduction, and more.
Paperback • $7.95 • 197 pages

THE HEALING POWER OF FAITH
A Study of Alternative Treatment Modalities
Will Ousler

Spiritual healing systems stand in contrast to traditional medicine and challenge it, and the new kinds of thinking they promote are symptoms of profound changes in our society and in ourselves. This book is a powerful testament to modern America's embrace of The Healing Power of Faith.
Paperback • 366 pages • $8.95

SEXUAL JOY THROUGH SELF-HYPNOSIS
Dr. Daniel L. Araoz and
Dr. Robert T. Bleck

This remarkable book teaches you how to overcome sexual problems that can arise through no fault of your own. Learn to overcome premature ejaculation and failure to reach orgasm; increase the intensity of your sexual experiences and gain an understanding of yourself and how your past may affect sexual expression.
Paperback • 222 pages • $9.95

HYPNOSPORT
Les Cunningham

An exciting work on the importance of subconcious reprogramming and mental training in athletic performance, Hypnosport is a major contribution to the field of sports conditioning and athletic motivation.
Paperback • $5.95 • 180 pages

TRANSFORMING THERAPY
A New Approach To Hypnotherapy
Gil Boyne

Here is a radically different approach to people-helping. Boyne has created a unique system that speaks simply yet eloquently to the issues of filling our deepest needs and realizing our highest potentials. Instead of attempting to penetrate the "mystery of trance" through the so called scientific methods, he focuses on solving problems by stimulating the inner creative mind.

"...A vivid dramatic, clinicial view into the innermost recesses of clients' emotional lives." –Robert F. Reid, Ph.D

Hardcover • 416 pages • $37.50 (includes free audio cassette)
Free audio cassette with purchase of Transforming Therapy, "Success Programming for the Hypnotherapist," a $12.50 value!

SELF HYPNOSIS AND OTHER MIND-EXPANDING TECHNIQUES
Charles Tebbetts

This book can make a wonderful difference in your life. Through easy- to-understand instructions, you will quickly learn the positive art of self-suggestion. Your guide is Charles Tebbetts, one of the foremost teachers of self-hypnosis. Among the areas covered: mastering the techniques of visualization and self-hypnosis; improve your health and sports performance; control addictions and other self-destructive emotions; relieve psychosomatic symptoms; improve your memory and concentration. Plus, you'll learn the unique benefits of meditation, biofeedback, faith healing and ESP.
Paperback • $7.95 • 141 pages

HYPNOSIS MOTIVATION CASSETTES
Self-Hypnosis *"POWER PROGRAMMING"*
by Gil Boyne, Certified Clinical Hypnotherapist

FILL IN AND MAIL... TODAY

WESTWOOD PUBLISHING COMPANY
700 S. Central Avenue, Dept. WW93
Glendale, CA 91204

USE YOUR CREDIT CARD AND ORDER BY PHONE
1-818-242-1159 or in California 1-800-89-HYPNO

Qty.	Description	Price	Total

*Up to $25.00 add $1.75; $25.01 to $60.00 add $2.75; $60.01 to $98.99 add $4.00; $99 and up ...FREE

**In California add 8.25% state sales tax.

Subtotal	
Postage & handling*	
Sales tax**	
TOTAL	

❑ Check enclosed for $_____, payable to Westwood Publishing
❑ Charge my ❑ Mastercard ❑ Visa ❑ American Express

Account No._____ Exp. Date_____

Signature_____

Your Name_____

Address_____

City/State/Zip_____

Daytime Telephone_____

GUARANTEE
You must be satisfied!
You get a 30-day, 100% money-back guarantee
on all books and audio casettes

Thank you for your order!